# 201 Diet Tips For Heart Patients

Dr. Bimal Chhajer, MD



FUSION BOOKS

©**Publisher :** Fusion Books
X-30, Okhla Industrial Area,
Phase-II, New Delhi-110020
Phone : 011-40712200
E-mail : wecare@diamondbooks.in
Website : www.diamondbooks.in
Edition : 2026
Printed By : Repro (India)

---

**201 Diet Tips For Heart Patients**
by ***DR. BIMAL CHHAJER*** M.D.

# INTRODUCTION

There are more than 6 crore (60 million) heart patients in India today and the number is growing fast towards 100 millions. About 28 lacs (2.8 millions) are likely to die every year from heart disease. Except for only 1-2% of these patients (who have valve defects or holes in the heart) all of these groups have blocked their tubes supplying the heart. These blockages grow from young age (15 years to 20 years) due to continuous deposition of fat on the inner side of the heart arteries. Once these blocks cover more than two thirds of the tubes (70% or more) – the complains start. The person thus becomes a heart patient.

**Out of the fifteen major reasons responsible for development of heart disease – at least ten are related to diet.**

There are probably five times more people, in this country, who are not yet heart patients but will develop the same in the coming years.

Out of the fifteen major reasons responsible for development of heart disease – at least ten are related to diet. The two major components of blockage are Cholesterol and Triglycerides (fats) – and both can be supplied to the body by out diet. Lack of fiber in the food, lack of anti-oxidants like vitamins A, C and E are directly related to heart disease. Diet also adversely affects high blood pressure, diabetes, obesity and LDL cholesterol. Some kinds of food can increase HDL Cholesterol and protect the heart from developing heart disease. Thus lack of HDL can be caused by wrong diet.

All these above facts suggest that Diet modification is a must in order to stop the progress of Coronary heart disease or to reverse the blockages that lead to this disease. Everyone agrees about this diet modification but the fact remains that most of the common people do not have adequate advice on this aspect from the cardiologists. Many of them go to the dieticians –but the result is a diet chart which can not be followed for rest of the life. After sometimes the heart patients stop following the chart and start developing the disease again.

As part of SAAOL Heart Program – where we train the heart patients to reverse these blockages in the coronary arteries- I found that all my participants have hundreds of questions on diet. They really want to know how the dieticians decide what to eat and what not to eat. They want to know the basis of calculation of calories, composition of diet and details about the fat contents of the food they love to eat. They want to know what foods are good and what are bad for their heart and why are they so. For the last ten years I have tried to answer them all – whatever they ask.

At this moment let me also remind you that diet only forms 30% of my recommendations for prevention and reversal of heart disease. Stress management, Yoga-Meditation, Education about the heart, regular walking and simultaneous intake of drugs are also very important part of my training program.

# WHY THIS BOOK?

For last one decade or so I have been answering on an average about 10 questions per day, asked by the heart patients I treat. When I answer one question they will be ready with the second. Doctor, Can I take salt? Which oil can I use for cooking? Can I apply oil on my body? Do you think olive oil is really good for the heart? Can I take polyunsaturated oil? Can I take Ghee? What if I take zero cholesterol oil?

SAAOL Heart Program which I and my colleagues developed in the last ten years or so have been extensively training people on diet, the diet which will help to prevent and reverse the heart disease, the diet which does not use any oil for cooking food. We found that just telling that do not put any oil is not sufficient. The patients must know why and why not. They must understand cholesterol and triglycerides and what are the differences between the two. To put them into practice we involved the lady members of the family and developed cooking classes for them.

In the initial phase the taste of our zero oil food was not at all good. It was like boiled food. But gradually we developed the art of cooking. This led to discovery of more than a thousand delicious dishes over the last 3-4 years. I have already published more than five books on "zero oil recipes" and they have become very popular. I also realized that heart patients and those who want to prevent heart disease look at diet as the most important culprit for the development of heart disease. They understand that diet is something that they can control to a great extent. Thus so many queries!

Then came the request from Mr.Narendra Verma of Diamond Pocket Books to provide them with a book, which answers all the queries of the heart patients. Thus this book.

In this book, you will find all the queries that you could think of about diet, answered in a very simple language. You must have asked such questions many times but you wouldn't have got such simple answers. But this book is simple and the answers are clear-cut. I hope you will like it.

# ACKNOWLEDGEMENT

I have been writing on diet for the last so many years. My diet advices to the heart patients are very simple "Do not use oil while you cook" and avoid high Cholesterol diet like, non-vegetarian food and high fat milk and milk products. Take calories appropriate to your weight. Add lot of fiber and antioxidants. This book has all my answers to the heart patients or those who want to prevent heart disease in future. I must thank all my patients (more that 7000 of them now) who spent three days with me while attending our SAAOL heart programme and bombarded me with all these questions. These questions were practical and covering their day-to-day life.

Amongst our dieticians (those who worked with me in the last ten years) I must thank all of them for helping me from time to time. Those who helped me especially for this book were Ms.Sapna Singh, Ms.Priyanka Rastogi and Ms. Shalini Rastogi. Priyanka did the early part of the text but Sapna helped me the most. It was she who wrote and rewrote all the answers discussed with me and went to the minutest details. She was very patient and worked hard clearing all the doubts. I must thank her for this book.

Others who need to be acknowledged for this book are Nand kishore who heads the DTP section of our organization, Dr.Arijit Chakravorty my assistant for the past few years, Dr.Subrato, Kishore, Bhupender, Vaibhav and Harish. Without their help this book would not have been possible.

# CONTENTS

## CEREALS AND PULSES

**MISCELLANEOUS**

# SAAOL HEART PROGRAMME

The SAAOL Heart Programme is an extensive three days training where a group of heart patients stay together to learn the science and art of living. Under the guidance of doctors, dieticians, yoga experts and trainer. The patients along with their spouses learn the perfect art of heart care.

This camp is organized in all the metros.In Delhi it is held every month and every three months in rest of the metros (Kolkata, Bangalore & Mumbai). By joining this camp you can avoid Bypass surgery, Angioplasty, Angiography and Heart attack.

For more details and free booklet write to:

**SAAOL Heart Center**
14/84-85, Vikram Vihar, Lajpat Nagar-IV,
Delhi-110024 Ph. 26235168, 26283098, Fax : 26212016
e mail: info@saaol.com   website: www.saaol.com

# SAAOL'S Zonal Centers

**North Zone : Delhi (Head Off.)**
*Mr. Harish*
SAAOL Heart Center,
14/84-85, Vikram Vihar,
Lajpat Nagar IV, New Delhi - 110024
Ph. : 26235168, 26283098, 26211908
Fax : 26212016
E-mail : info@saaol.com

**South Zone : Bangalore**
*Mr. S.S. Prasad*
25, S.P. Road, Off. 4th Temple Street,
Malleswaram, Bangalore - 560003.
Ph. : 56993797, 23462869
Mobile : 36736554
E-mail : ssprasaad@yahoo.com

**West Zone : Mumbai**
*Mr. Deepak Dalal*
B- 301, Gold Mist, Thakur Complex,
Kandivili (E), Mumbai - 400101
Ph. : 56995378, 28543088
Fax : 28544217

**East Zone : Kolkata**
*Mr. Praveen*
65/4A, Flat No : 1A,
Sarat Bose Road, Kolkata-25
Ph.: 30930329 Mobile: 32570713.

# THE PRESENT DAY TREATMENT OF HEART DISEASE

The number of heart patients in India has increased at a very high speed in the last three decades basically because of worsening lifestyle. Some of the major causes are high fat content of Indian diet (e.g. Excessive use of oil, cream, milk and milk products), increased mechanization and lack of physical activity (e.g. cars, telephones, washing machines, gadgets, lack of time to do exercise and so on) and increased stress (e.g. competition due to increased population, breaking down of joint family structure, increased expenditure at the face of stagnant income). These causes alongwith the lack of education about heart disease and smaller factors have created blockages of Cholesterol and Triglycerides inside the heart arteries of millions of people. The result is enormous loss of life, increased medical expenditure of millions of families and loss of livelihood for those suffering from this fatal disease.

Frankly speaking, the doctors dealing with heart disease (the Cardiologists and Cardiac surgeons) have remained silent spectators in this worsening scenario. Without seriously working on the causes of heart disease (correction of food habits, education of heart patients on causes of heart disease) they found out temporary measures, which might help themselves economically. Hospitals started CCUs(coronary care units), increased the number of Angioplasties and Bypass surgeries and patients were given the idea that these are the only ways to solve their heart disease. The result was that the number of patients grew. The number of heart hospitals gradually also increased. A vicious cycle gradually came into existence.

The process of Angioplasty actually involves clearing of the heart tubes by pressing the fatty materials on the sides by using balloons and protecting the collapse by using stents (which are nothing but perforated hollow tubes). The real cause of the blockages the ongoing deposit of fatty materials and the reactions of the body to the stents rebuild the blockages within the span of few months to years. The cost of these procedures have increased enormously by three to five folds in the last few years without really adding much of benefit.

The Bypass surgery on the other hand is a mutilating operation, which leaves two to three big scars in the body besides hosts of complications. The additional tubes stitched to the heart make a temporary channel which flows blood to the heart muscles. The food habits remaining same, bad lifestyle prevailing the new channels start closing the day it was stitched to the heart. Usually it takes five years to close these tubes to the extent that it causes the problems again. The third option is to continue the medicines, which give a relief to the patient from chest pain and symptoms. The causes of the disease remaining same the blockage gradually grows and soon the patient suffers from a heart attack. The heart hospitals keep the ICCUs ready for these people to get admitted.

The gist is that the medical science/cardiology science is heading towards a doom. The real solution for heart disease will never come in this way. We have to look for a new approach. An approach, which is rational, based on simple common sense. And this approach should analyze the causes of heart disease and guide the patients to get rid of the causative factors. This will stop the disease from growing. The medical science is now agreeing that it is possible to even reverse the heart disease and the blockages if the causes are taken care of in a very accurate way. Thanks to recent research studies by Dean Ornish and other medical scientists.

SAAOL (Science and art of Living) Heart Programme is aimed exactly to do the reversal of heart disease. We developed this heart care programme where the treatment of heart disease is originating from the rectification of the underlying causes of heart disease. The training programme educates the heart disease on diet; yoga, meditation, exercise programme, stress management; control of cholesterol, blood pressure, diabetes, weight and all the possible ways to help the heart to heal itself. These training programmes are held regularly all over the country (Delhi in North, Mumbai in West, Kolkata in East and Bangalore in South).

# HEART AND ITS FUNCTIONS

The human heart is a small muscular organ situated in the center of the chest, tilted to the left side. In size, it is roughly that of a clenched fist and weighs about 350 gms. As it is such an important and delicate organ, it is protected by the chest bone or sternum and ribs in front.

## How Heart Works?

**Heart beats about 72 times and amounts to about 2,500,000,000 beats in a person's life span of 70 years. It circulates about 5 ltrs of blood every minute.**

The heart is mostly made up of a strong muscle tissue called the myocardium and it works continuously like a tireless pump, quietly day and night, throughout a man's life time. It beats about 72 times a minute, and if we calculate the number of minutes in our life time, it amounts to about 2,500,000,000 beats in a person's life-span of 70 years. It circulates about 5 litres of blood every minute, amounting to about 700 million litres of blood in a lifetime. During physical exercise and mental stress, this function can increase up to 6 fold or even more. Thus, making heart the most efficient pump known to mankind. In spite of all the advances made

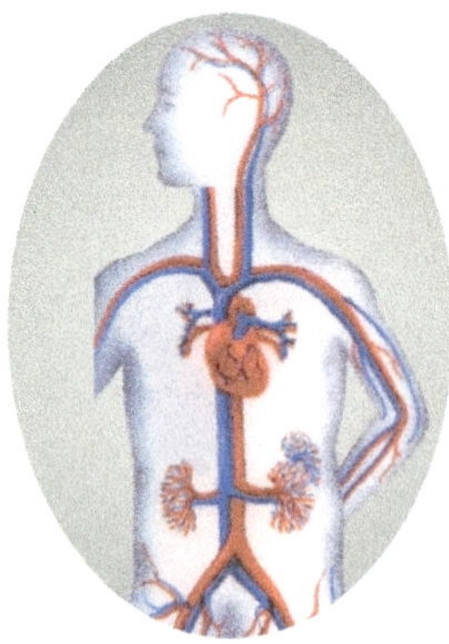

in fields of science and medical technology, nobody has been able to artificially replicate such a pump.

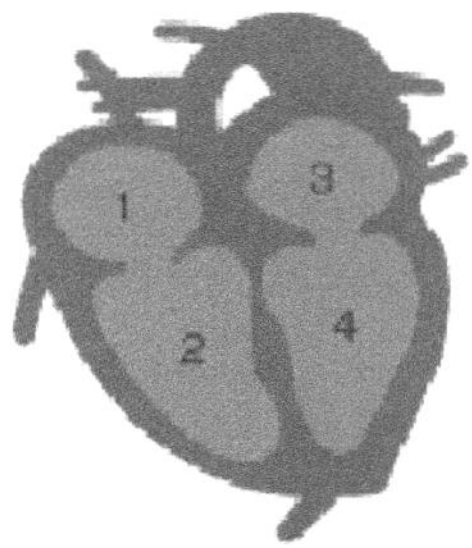

The Four Chambers of Heart

Internally, the heart is divided into 4 chambers, and has four major valves. The upper two chambers are called the atria and the lower two, the ventricles. The right atria receives impure or deoxygenated blood (blood which has been deprived of it's oxygen content by tissues) via veins from the whole body, this blood goes to the right ventricle which contracts and pumps it through the pulmonary arteries (blood vessels connecting the heart to the lungs) to the lungs where it is oxygenated. The oxygenated or purified blood from the lungs goes to the left atria via the pulmonary veins (the only veins in the human body to carry oxygenated blood) and into the left ventricle which contracts and pumps it with tremendous force throughout the entire body and supplies it to the billions of tissues which make up the human body. In this manner blood circulates in the human body.

**Functions**

The function of the heart is to supply blood and essential nutrients to the whole body. The body uses oxygen to stay alive. Besides supplying blood, oxygen and nutrition to all parts of the body, the circulatory system also regulates body's internal temperature, distributes hormones and removes the harmful by-products of metabolism, including a host of other functions.

List of the functions of the heart

- Supplying blood to entire body.
- Supplying Oxygen and nutrients (digested food particles that we eat) to the whole body and to billions of cells in the body

- Giving Vitamins and Minerals to cells of the body, without which they cannot survive.
- Carrying or pulling blood back to the heart and sending the same to the lungs for a refill of oxygen.
- Help in distribution of hormones, neuro chemicals from one part of body to another.
- Help taking the waste materials to the kidney for purification of the blood. The kidney extracts waste from blood.

# WHAT IS A HEART DISEASE?

> **When the blockages exceeds beyond 70% it leads to coronary heart disease or angina.**

Coronary heart disease (constitutes more than 95% of heart patients) can be called as the **Disease of Ignorance,** as it develops due to the lack of knowledge. Human body is one of the best machines in the world and if maintained properly it cannot develop a snag. Heart disease is actually a result of long period of mis-management of heart by wrong lifestyle. With the wrong food, excessive fats and cholesterol, lack of control of diabetes and high blood pressure, less exercise, smoking and consumption of tobacco and excessive stress- people start developing blockages in the heart tubes. Starting is always from zero. Repetitions of the same, year after year, the blockages grow until the blockages reach the range of about 70%. And that's when the heart disease is diagnosed.

Heart disease mostly refers to the disease which is caused by accumulation of fat and cholesterol in the arteries (blood carrying tubes in the walls of the heart). It is because this particular disease accounts for more than 95% of heart ailments. This means that out of 10 patients with heart ailments more than 9 will have obstruction in the blood flow to the muscles of the heart.

This disease of blockage of the heart arteries is medically called **"Coronary Heart Disease (CHD)"**. Over the years the same disease has been referred to, by different names, by different people in different regions. The most common of these names is **"Angina"**. Angina means a pain on the left side of the chest often radiating to the left arm. Since this pain is commonly found in 80 % of the people having Coronary Heart Disease, angina also became the most common name.

A little less known name of the same disease is **"Ischemia"-** (Shortage of oxygen). All the problems of the CHD occur due to shortage of oxygen (of course due to the blockage in the tubes supplying blood to the heart muscles.). "Ischemia" is a more scientific term. CHD is also referred to as the **Ischemic Heart Disease or IHD.**

# HOW THE BLOCKAGE TAKES PLACE?

When the heart supplies the blood to the aorta (the main artery for the body) it retains two branches for its own supply. The muscles of the heart which have to contract continuously obviously need a continuous supply of blood. This blood brings food and oxygen- which gives it power in the form of Calories.

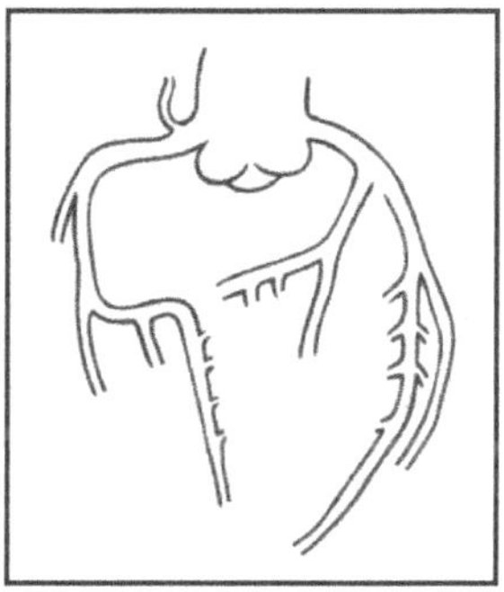

The Coronary Arteries

These tubes are called coronary tubes, because when they divide and re-divide, they look like a crown on the head of a king. There are two main tubes that form this crown.

Out of the two one is on the right side, called the Right Coronary Artery or RCA which has a diameter of 5 mm. It gives off, a series of branches as it goes down and circles around the right side of the heart and proceeds as the PDA. The tube can be divided into three parts - proximal third, middle third and distal third.

The branch to the heart in the left is called the Left main (LM) which immediately divides into two branches.

The first branch, the Left Anterior Descending (LAD), is so named as it supplies to the front (called Anterior in medical language) of the heart and goes down (called Descending in medical language), supplies the blood through numerous branches to the heart muscles. It gives some branches in the right direction, called the septal branches (named as $S_1$, $S_2$, $S_3$ and so on) and some on the left direction called Diagonal branches ($D_1$, $D_2$, $D_3$ and so on). For purpose of easy description, this artery (LAD) can also be divided into three parts – proximal third, middle third and distal third. The LAD is bigger than RCA in size and is more important as it supplies main part of the "Chamber four or Left Ventricle".

The second branch on the left side of the heart is called Left Circumflex (LCx) as it circles down the circumference of the heart on the left side. This is little smaller than the RCA in size.

The circumflex artery gives branches to supply all the areas in the back of the left side of the heart. Some of the branches of this tube are called Obtuse Marginal and are expressed as $OM_1$, $OM_2$, and $OM_3$ and so on.

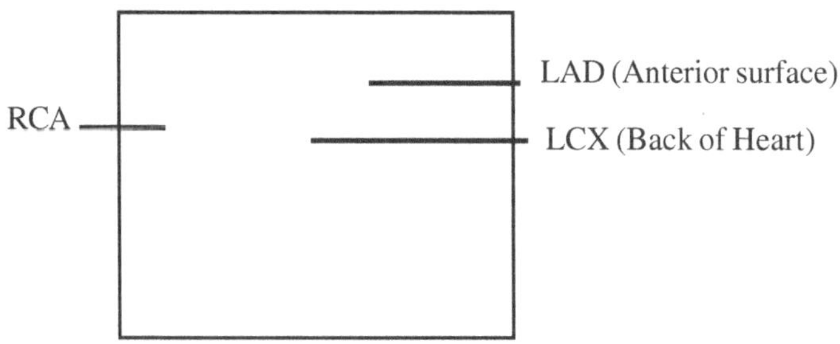


The Coronary Arteriesand their branches (A-P View)

# HOW TO RECOGNIZE HEART DISEASE?

Angina is the sensation of heaviness or pain in left side of the chest which typically radiates to left arm. It may be associated with sweating, choking sensation and breathlessness.

Angina pain usually occurs on sudden excitement, anxiety, climbing stairs, walking, bathing or during any stressful activity. Angina is specially felt on minimal exertion after heavy meals. The symptoms are relieved on taking rest or a Sorbitrate (nitro-glycerine) tablet below the tongue. This pain is never an excruciating pain in nature and does not stay for a long time. If these two occur then it indicates a heart attack, medically known as Myocardial Infarction.

Recognition of angina depends on the patient's knowledge about the disease and physical activity. If one performs heavy physical activity from time to time (where the heart rate is raised beyond 120-130/minute) one can identify angina early. People who do not physically exert themselves feel and recognize angina quite late, because they never reach a higher heart rate. Many such physically inactive persons sometimes get fatal heart attacks which may even result in death, simply because they could not identify angina and take care.

Angina does not occur at blockages of 40 to 50% which is widely prevalent. If it occurs, it is more likely to be precipitated by a sudden episode of coronary artery spasm which is the most common manifestation of stress.

**Common symptoms of angina are :**

1. **Chest pain**: The pain of Angina may have its severity from mild to severe, whereas the pain of a Heart attack is very severe. It usually occurs in center of the chest and radiates to left arm but at times may even radiate to the right arm, shoulders or the lower jaws. The pain usually lasts for 5 to 10 minutes.

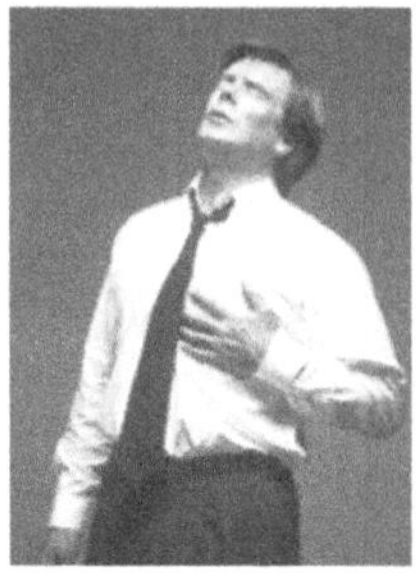

2. **Breathlessness** or **Shortness of Breath.**
3. **Sweating.**
4. **Nausea** (sensation of vomiting) and **vomiting**
5. **Dizziness** and **Fainting.**
6. **Pain** or **Heaviness** in chest especially after heavy meals.
7. **Choking** sensation in the throat.
8. **Heaviness** or **Tightness in the chest** or upper abdomen.
9. **Weakness** and easy **Fatigability**.

# WHAT IS HEART ATTACK?

Angina appears when the blockage becomes 70% or more. These blockages always develop under a membrane called internal membrane (Intima), which gets stretched gradually with the increase in blockage.

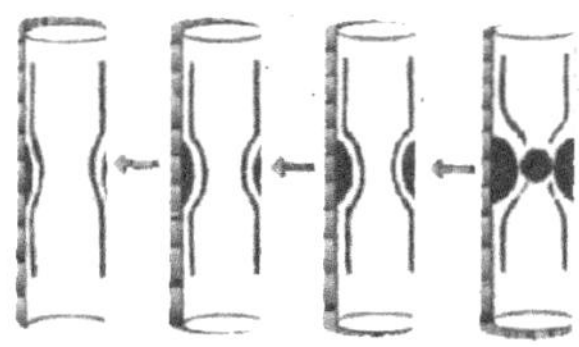

Finally one day this membrane ruptures (breaks off) which is followed by clotting of blood, changing the block now to 100%. This cuts off the blood supply entirely leading to a Heart Attack.

This 100% block leads to severe pain, sweating and ultimately some area of the heart muscle dies leading to a permanent damage.

Heart Attack or Myocardial Infarction (medically called MI or Coronary Thrombosis) is the consequence of the complete obstruction of blood supply to a part of the heart muscles. This occurs due to a 100% blockage in any of the coronary arteries or their branches. The heart muscles are completely deprived of their blood and oxygen supply which leads to death.

The severity of the heart attack would depend on how much area of the heart muscle is actually involved. It is mild, if only 5 to 10 % area is involved and most of the patients survive. But if the dead area is more than 30 to 40 % of the heart muscles, the attack is considered severe, and if not managed properly and immediately, can even lead to death.

**Myocardial Infarction (medically called MI or Coronary Thrombosis) is the consequence of the complete obstruction of blood supply to a part of the heart muscles. This occurs due to a 100% blockage**

Almost all the heart attacks are sudden in onset and the cause is a rupture of the growing blockages. The blockages are usually covered by a thin membrane called *Intimal* membrane, which also keep the deposits intact. This elastic membrane gets more and more stretched as more and more fatty deposits occur. But if the fatty deposits continue below this permeable membrane, one day the time will come, when the membrane cannot stretch further and breaks off. This leads to the formation of a clot or thrombus inside the tube, closing the lumen completely. This completes the process of heart attack. The area of the myocardium (heart muscles) which gets the blood through the closed artery, dies - in the event of no blood supply.

Heart attack, often occurs after a heavy meal full of fat, after sudden anger or excessive sorrow or grief or excessive stress. Heart attacks occur more frequently in the early mornings. Heart attacks also occur during the process of Angiography and Angioplasty when the catheter or balloon is inflated and completely blocks the lumen of the coronary artery or breaks off the blockage by mechanical means.

The diagram and few paragraphs above, give the clue to prevention of heart attacks. The simple message is "Do not create more blockages. If you can reduce it, heart attack would never occur."

It is like a bundle of notes being guarded by a rubber band. If you keep on putting more and more notes inside the rubber band one day the rubber band has to snape due to excessive stretching. This is the situation of a heart attack where the membrane also breaks off. Now if you stop putting more notes, the rubber band will not break. Further, if you start taking out one or two notes from the bundle everyday, the rubber band will never break.

The same principle applies in prevention of heart attack. Control of all the risk factors of heart disease by adequate change in the lifestyle can prevent heart attacks. The following are the expected parameters to prevent heart attacks:

1. Cholesterol 130 to 160 mg/dl
2. Triglycerides 60 to 120 mg/dl
3. HDL Cholesterol 40 to 60 mg/dl
4. Blood glucose (Fasting) 70 to 100 mg/dl
5. Blood Glucose (PP) below 140 mg/dl
6. Blood Pressure 120/80 mmHg
7. Maximum permissible exercises
8. Body weight in proportion to height
9. Stop smoking completely
10. Control stress
11. Oil/Ghee in food is banned completely
12. Consume salads and fruits in plenty
13. Restrict consumption of milk and milk products
14. Avoid meat of any kind.

# RISK FACTORS FOR DEVELOPING HEART DISEASE

Coronary Heart Disease (CHD) or Coronary Artery Disease (CAD) or Ischemic Heart Disease (IHD) is one of the leading causes of morbidity and mortality throughout the world. It is on a constant rise now in India too. The main cause of this disease is deposition of cholesterol and fat in the inner smooth lining of the blood vessels (coronary arteries - supplying blood to the heart), resulting in blockages and obstruction of blood flow through them.

Certain conditions and life-style habits are now recognized and documented to be responsible for the deposition of cholesterol and fat in blood vessels as well as the increased rate at which they are being deposited, these are referred to as Risk Factors.

Risk factors are the reasons which lead to or aggravate the deposition of cholesterol or fat in the coronary arteries. All the factors which are important in the development of coronary heart disease, they have been classified into 2 categories:

**1). Modifiable Risk Factors:**

In this group comes those risk factors which can be altered and prevented so that the further progress of heart disease can be arrested.

**2). Non-Modifiable Risk Factors:**

There are three risk factors which cannot be altered such as age, sex and heredity.

Classification of Risk Factors predispoing to Coronary Heart Disease

**Modifiable Risk Factors**

1) Stress
2) High blood cholesterol level
3) High blood Triglyceride level
4) Low blood HDL level
5) Lack of antioxidants in the diet
6) High blood pressure
7) Diabetes mellitus
8) Obesity or Overweight
9) Sedentary life-style or lack of physical activity
10) Smoking or tobacco consumption.
11) Alcohol consumption.

**Non-Modifiable Risk Factors**

1) Age
2) Sex
3) Heredity

### 1. Blood level of Cholesterol:

Blood Cholesterol is one of the most known risk factors of Coronary Heart Disease. Previously Cholesterol was supposed to be the most important cause of Heart Artery Blockages but with more and more research data coming in, it has become one of the first three risk factors.

Cholesterol is a type of fat particle present in the blood in small quantities. This waxy particle is made up of a single chain of fatty acid with 27 carbon atoms. The structure is so complex that this fatty acid is rotated in four rings - in combination called Cyclo- pentano-perhydro-phenantherene ring. It is one of the most decorated molecules - known to the medical science.

Cholesterol has very important functions in the body - as it forms a part of the cell wall, nerve coverings and the brain cells. We cannot imagine life without this molecule. So important is the requirement of Cholesterol in the body that the liver has a manufacturing capacity of the minimum amount of Cholesterol required by the body.

But if this molecule is present in more than adequate quantity in the body or blood, the excess can be deposited to create coronary blockages. Not only heart is affected; high cholesterol can also get deposited inside the brain arteries, leg arteries and also in the skin below the eyes.

Cholesterol carried in the blood is in free form, which is very dangerous and it can be also carried in combination of proteins (known as lipo-proteins). There is a strong relationship of blood level of free Cholesterol and rate of deposition of blockages in the heart arteries.

Previously it was presumed that a Cholesterol level of 250mg/100ml of blood is normal and safe. This was about 20 years back. After a lot of further research, it was found that a level less than 220mg/100ml was okay in the next ten years. But the latest scientific research has now proved that any level more than 200 mg/100ml is definitely not good. The normal range of this fat is now considered between 130 and 200 mg/100ml of blood. SAAOL Heart Programme recommends a level of Cholesterol lower than 160mg/100ml of blood to achieve optimum results. It is quite a common sense that we should try for the lowest of the normal range if the option is given.

The blood levels of Cholesterol are high in those people whose diet is rich in Cholesterol. The food that contain high Cholesterol are Egg Yolk, meat of any kind (Mutton, Beef, Chicken, Pork- both red Meat and white Meat, Fish). Another rich source is Milk and its products like Ghee, Cream, Butter, Ice Cream, Chocolates, Paneer, Curd etc. This becomes the culprit in vegetarians, who depend heavily on milk. Any other fat, especially the saturated fatty acids are used in the liver to manufacture Cholesterol.

Cholesterol is mostly deposited in the heart arteries, after it is converted into LDL Cholesterol, the so-called Bad "Lowdensity Lipo-protein Cholesterol"

SAAOL recommends very low Cholesterol (130-160mg/100ml) in the blood. The total intake of Cholesterol in the diet of a person should be as low as 10mg/day.

Regular physical exercise, stress management, stopping of smoking can also lead to lowering of the Cholesterol in the blood, besides control of diet.

**2. Blood level of Triglycerides:**

The other fat, besides Cholesterol, that had gained importance in the latest series of research studies is Triglycerides-being a major cause of heart disease. Almost all the fats that we eat in our food are nothing but Triglycerides. This is probably the other name for OILS. Triglycerides also form a part of the blockage.

Tri means three and Glycerides come from Glycerol. Triglyceride is a combination of one Glycerol molecule with three fats (or fatty acids). In other words, three chains of fat molecules (units) when attached to one Glycerol can constitute Triglycerides. These three chains of fatty acids, depending on the number of Hydrogen atoms that they contain, can be saturated, mono unsaturated or poly unsaturated. Almost all kinds of oil is 100% fat irrespective of any combination of these three kinds of fat. It is through the bad and unethical advertisements, for promoting their products that the oil-companies have created an impression that Triglycerides are good for the heart disease (which is interpreted as "helping to cure heart disease by the patients".

The normal Triglycerides are 60 – 160 mg/dl. SAAOL recommends bringing it down to < 130 mg/dl for reversal.

### 3. Low HDL Cholesterol

HDL cholesterol is the so called "good" cholesterol and can be measured from a fasting blood sample. It has a very high affinity to bind cholesterol and can remove cholesterol from the blockages.

HDL cholesterol level in the blood should be maintained above 40 mg per 100 ml of blood to prevent heart disease. Indians are known to have low HDL cholesterol and it is often seen that the average HDL cholesterol in Indians is below 40 mg per 100 ml of blood.

### 4. High Blood Pressure

The normal blood pressure in adults is between 100/60 to 140/90 mm Hg. If the blood pressure is consistently more than 140/90 on two or more separate occasions, it is called **High Blood Pressure** or **Hypertension**. It is a very common disease and about 20% to 30% of adults suffer from Hypertension all over the world, but a majority of people are not even aware that they have this disease because it does not produce any symptoms in a vast number of them. This is why this disease has been corrcctly called the "silent killer". High blood pressure puts an extra strain on the heart and the arteries supplying blood to the other organs of the body. Many diseases are caused by High blood pressure such as heart-attacks, heart-failure, kidney-failure, stroke (damage to the brain), and damage to the eyes. Higher the blood-pressure, greater are the chances of getting the above diseases, mainly heart attacks.

High blood pressure can be classified as **Mild, Moderate** and **Severe**. It is also one of the major causes of deposition of cholesterol and fat in the coronary arteries. It damages the endothelial lining of arteries, making them more prone to fat deposition. Besides a high intake of salt, psychological stress is also implied as important causes of high blood pressure.

## 5. Diabetes Mellitus

The normal levels of blood sugar in a fasting person is between 80-120 mg%. If the fasting level of blood sugar is more than 110 mg%, or after meals more than 160 mg%, it is called diabetes or high blood-sugar. In diabetic patients, sugar can be detected in the urine also. Patients with diabetes have a higher chances of development of coronary blockages. They also get several other diseases like kidney-damage, as well as damage to the nerves and eyes. Patients with diabetes are usually obese, have high blood pressure and high blood cholesterol levels, all responsible for blockages. Heart attack occur at a younger age in severe diabetics. The symptoms of diabetes are increased thirst, increased urination and weight loss, but in some there may be no symptoms at all. Control of diabetes is must for heart patients. India has a very high number of diabetic patients.

## 6. Obesity or Overweight

If the weight of a person is more than the upper limit of weight for that age and sex, he is called obese or a fat person. People who eat too much fat and do not exercise put on weight. There are standard charts available from which one can find out whether one is overweight or obese. Obese individuals have greater chances of getting heart diseases. They have increased chances of getting high blood pressure and diabetes and thereby blockages. Obesity can be prevented by eating low caloric food, avoiding fats, avoiding too much sugar, and undertaking regular physical exercise. Fat people remain inactive and are also made fun at sometimes. Therefore, they tend to develop excessive mental tensions resulting in hypertension and heart attacks. The chances of getting heart attacks increase by15 times for obese people as compared to lean and thin individuals. SAAOL recommends a slow but sustained reduction of weight in obese patients. A reduction of 2-3 kg per month is ideal.

### 7. Antioxidants and fibre:

Antioxidants are agents which oppose oxidation. Oxidation is the process which is damaging by virtue of its nature to cause degeneration. In the circulating blood both cholesterol and oxygen are present. It is the oxidation of cholesterol which leads to its deposition which builds up the blockages. Example of oxidation can be best understood by understanding the rusting of iron. Iron when exposed to air forms rust which is due to oxidation of iron. So antioxidants oppose this process and retard or prevent degeneration. Examples are Vitamin A, C, E and minerals like Selenium, Calcium and Zinc.

Fibre is present in all the vegetables and their covers and fruits. Firstly they do not have any calories because they increase the bulk of food that we eat and get excreted in the stool. They also make the bowels smoother. Since they are the mesh work of fibers. They entrap the fat particles which are mixed in the food. Hence they also get excreted out.

# MEDICAL TESTS TO CONFIRM HEART DISEASE

There are various tests, available for the confirmation of coronary heart disease.

1. **Physical Checkup** - Before any other tests are ordered complete physical examination of the patient is performed that involves measuring blood pressure and pulse rate. Fresh lipid profile as well as blood sugar tests are also ordered.

2. **ECG (Electrocardiogram)** - is one of the safest tests available. The cardiologists use it most widely. Changes in the ECG are confirmatory of heart disease.

3. **TMT (Treadmill Test)** - is done only when Electrocardiogram does not provide any conclusive evidence of Coronary Artery Disease or gives equivocal findings. This is one of the highly reliable non-invasive tests for the confirmation of Coronary Artery Disease.

4. **ECHO Cardiogram** - is usually done to find out the pumping power of the heart. It also gives good information about the walls of the heart.

5. **Angiography** - In this test a long wire is used to fill up the blocked tubes of the heart with a radio opaque dye, and thereafter, approximate percentages of blockages are reported. This is a test which carries a definite risk in itself, inspite of being costly and imprecise. Only those who are keen to go for angioplasty or bypass surgery should go ahead with this test.

# HOW TO PREVENT AND REVERSE HEART DISEASE?

**Saaol Heart Programme comprises of Yoga, Meditation, Heart Rejuvenating exercises, diet and meditation**

The most rational solution to coronary heart disease lies in a permanent process which not only arrests progress of the blockage but also reverses the same. The blockage has gradually occurred over a period of time consisting of several years, as the cholesterol from blood flows through the coronary arteries and get deposited (due to the risk factors) in the arterial wall. These deposits are mostly soft mass of fat with connective tissues and are in a reversible phase. It has now been proved that cholesterol and fat are easily dissoluble in the blood, and can be picked up from the blockages if we can create an ideal situation for this process to occur.

It is essential to create this ideal situation SAAOL Heart Programme helps and trains people to create these ideal situations; cutting down of all the risk factors at a time with carefully selected set of Yogasanas, Meditation; a perfect practically possible stress management programme; complete education and understanding of coronary heart disease; cessation of tobacco intake, smoking and food awareness-cooking training - directs one to a perfect lifestyle which can reverse the blockages. All of these have to be done under the guidance of Cardiologists, Doctors, Dieticians, and Yoga Masters in order to avoid complications - which are easy to develop for heart patients.

All heart patients know a little bit about some preventive measures, and they try doing these without much accuracy and consistency making unsuccessful efforts and finally submitting to the surgical treatment. Had it not been happening, none of these patients would go to a hospital in cases of emergency.

**The SAAOL Heart Programme** has developed this expertise over the last decade after a lot of experimentation and efforts. Each and every patient joining the programme in initial phase has helped the programme to improve gradually. Heart attacks and other complications have been extremely low.

**The SAAOL Heart Programme** is not magic - it cannot perform like a magician or God who would remove the blockage in a moment. It takes atleast two weeks to see first sign of improvement. The improvement will also depend on efforts put in by patients, his/her age, stage of blockage, co-operation of family members and so on. We now have some Angiographies of our patients, done after attending the **SAAOL Heart Programme** which proves that blockages can be reversed.

Reading books is a good way of learning but cannot substitute a practical training. Otherwise, the bookshops would have been chock full selling treatment programmes only. Books contain hundreds of pages - some of them very important but most of them are not relevant to patients and difficult to understand. It is much more difficult to translate and put the written word into practise. If this were not so, then every patient could have become doctor by buying medical books - and learning whatever doctors know.

Nevertheless, what helps definitely is the fact that when you have someone who can give you the information you need - not so voluminous that you don't comprehend it at all and definitely not less so that you do not learn at all.

# DR. DEAN ORNISH
# THE REAL PROOF

Little was thought that this particular second-year medical student of the Baylor College of Medicine, Houston, who would one day be one of the greatest pioneers in the most effective and logical treatments developed for the cure and reversal of heart disease, America's No. 1 killer. This American killer disease is rapidly growing to considerable potential in our country.

Dr. Dean Ornish, born and bred in Dallas, received his preliminary education from a public school. His father being a dentist by profession was quite content by the thought that some day his son would follow in his footsteps. Dr. Ornish joined the Rice University at Houston and discovered that he was no longer the brightest student. So depressed was he that he even contemplated suicide, but as fate would have it an episode of glandular fever gave him the chance to reconsider, and thus rendering on to us a pioneer in the Reversal of Coronary Heart Disease and salvation from it.

Like many others of his generation in 1972, he too sought the enlightenment of the Orient and under the wings of his Guru, the honorable Swami Sachidanand he succeeded in touching his inner self and realized that less he needed success, the less strained he felt. This led him to suspect the connection between depression and heart. And in 1977 he started researching the causes of heart disease and factors that could possibly bring about its reversal. His explorations began while he was still a 2nd year medical student, and for a very long time no one could see the potential in his work. His seniors and critics dismissed him as young, inexperienced and foolishly idealistic. While he was still in his third year of medical school he received his first big break-through. He was introduced to Henry Groppe, an oil business consultant, who had a firm interest in preventive medicine. Dr. Dean Ornish formulated a plan of Life Style changes which had 4 major disciplines, all aiming at an integrated attack on heart disease and its reversal:

1. Stress management which would comprise YOGA, MEDITATION, IMAGERY and BREATHING EXERCISES all together for the duration of not more than an hour a day.
2. Light AEROBIC EXERCISE which would usually be quite convenient and half an hour's walk.
3. He would ask his patients to stop smoking.
4. And to adhere to a strictly VEGETARIAN DIET extremely low in fat content.

Dr. Ornish's life style plan is simple and easy to understand and follow. His approach of combating heart disease and its reversal produced remarkable results. Truly we can say that "the greatest truths are the simplest ones". And in 1989 he started publishing data showing that his "Firehouse gang" as he preferred to call them, who were at one time very seriously ill were in fact improving. The attention of the world was soon focussed on his work and soon invitations to medical conferences began pouring in. Currently he is also receiving grants from many international organisations including the U.S. National Institute of Health (NIH). Dr. Dean Ornish's program recently got a new support from a very reputed insurance company "Medicare" of USA. They have agreed to send 1800 patients in the next 3 years to Dean Ornish's Program at the cost of $7200 per patient. With this the company will save a huge amount of money. The acknowledgment of tremendous potential of this humble man's work will one day lead us to the development of a far better and more advanced medical therapeutic approach to the cure and reversal of heart disease from which every one can benefit.

Dr. Ornish published his first report as early as in 1979. In 1983 in a report published in JAMA (Journal of American Medical Association) he showed lowering of all risk factors of heart disease in patients who followed the lifestyle advised by him. He showed that pumping power of the heart also increased in his patients. In 1990, Dr. Ornish gained wide recognition to his work after he showed Angiographically that a reversal of arterial blockages did occur in patients enlisted in his program. This scientific report featured in the most prestigious medical journal - the Lancet. He was then frequently quoted in Newsweek, USA news, Reader's Digest, Span etc. - some of the most widely recognized magazines in the world. He showed all the proof of reversal when he used the latest medical gadget "PET Scan" to prove his reversal theory. This scientific report was again published in the year 1995 by the JAMA (Journal of American Medical Association). The whole scientific world had to at last stop and listen. The theory became widely accepted in USA and the world. Today, Dr. Ornish offers his reversal programs in eight major hospitals in USA including Harward Medical School, Boston and Beth Israel Hospital, New York City.

Dr. Dean Ornish's results are now widely accepted. The latest text books of cardiology have also begun to include a separate chapter on Reversal of Heart Disease. The latest edition (1997) of the most reputed text book of cardiology, one of the most popular and voluminous books in the medical sciences - Braunwald's text book writes elaborately about how Dr. Dean Ornish proved that blockages can be reversed.

# WHAT IS SAAOL?

**The SAAOL -** Science And Art Of Living established in 1995 is the most comprehensive cardiac rehabilitation and Heart Disease Reversal Programme in India. Till now 6000 patients have been benefited from SAAOL Heart Program with a success rate of 98%.

**Purpose:** To reduce the risk of heart disease through complete change in lifestyle that includes diet modification, stress management, exercise, yoga, meditation, health education and counselling. Our primary goal is to foster independence: enabling individuals to self-monitor their activities and to take primary responsibility for healthier lifestyle behaviour and risk factor reduction. In practical terms, the SAAOL offers the following:

1. Lifestyle Modification
2. Medical evaluation/Drug treatment
3. Risk factor evaluation/stratification
4. Exercise prescription based on individual functional capacity
5. Personalized exercise programme
6. Education and support for risk factor modification
7. Dietary counselling
8. Smoking Cessation
9. Stress Management
10. Yoga
11. Meditation

# REVERSAL - THE MOST RATIONAL TREATMENT

The blockage occurs due to the slow but steady deposits of fatty material – cholesterol and Triglycerides inside the arteries of the heart and our modern lifestyle has allowed it to grow. The most rational solution to coronary heart disease lies in adopting a permanent process, which not only arrests the progress of the blockages but also reverses the same. In order to slowly reverse the blockages an ideal body environment is required in which cholesterol and fat can be picked up from the blockages.

SAAOL Heart Program helps people to create that ideal body environment by training them on how to cut down all the risk factors simultaneously, which includes complete education and understanding of coronary heart disease carefully practicing selected set of yogasanas, meditation, a perfect & practically possible stress management programme, cessation of tobacco intake or smoking and a food awareness that consists zero oil cooking training. Thus, it directs one into a perfect lifestyle, which can reverse the blockages. All these have to be done under the guidance of Cardiologists, Dieticians, Yoga Experts in order to avoid complication – which are easy to develop for heart patients.

Hence, the ideal and the most scientific treatment of CHD would naturally be controlling or modifying risk factors for the development of heart disease.

**Physical**

1. Developing regular physical activity and exercise regimen.
2. Maintaining a normal bodyweight.

**Behavioural**

1. Properly managing stress, anxiety, worry and anger.
2. Saying no to smoking and tobacco related products.
3. Avoiding faulty food habits, eg. Excess of milk and milk products, non-vegetarian food etc.
4. Avoiding intake of visible oil in food.
5. Avoiding alcohol consumption.

**Medical**

1. Maintaining normal blood pressure
2. Maintaining normal serum Cholesterol
3. Maintaining normal serum Triglycerides
4. Maintaining normal HDL Cholesterol
5. Maintaining normal blood sugar

If Heart disease has to be prevented, these factors should be properly controlled. The development of CHD is closely linked to three factors, first of all, the level of increasing stress in daily life is very important. Secondly, the level of decreasing physical activity and lastly, faulty dietary patterns pursued all are equally important.

## Physical Activity

Patients with varying severity of disease and belonging to different age groups have different levels of physical fitness. Thus, the amount of exercise performed by the heart patient should be according to his or her requirement. The exercise regimen is constructed in such a manner so as to open up the collaterals (small tubes which are closed and take over the functions once the normal arteries of the heart gets clogged) through appropriate cardiovascular conditioning. Yoga, Meditation, Kayotsarg and Health Rejuvenating Exercises (HRE) form an integral component of such a regimen.

## Dietary Habits

As CAD occurs because of the development of blockages (deposits of Cholesterol and Triglycerides) present in the three major tubes. Unless and until we stop the supply of these fats and oils from outside, we can never get rid of the disease. Hence the food that is to be consumed by the heart patients should be absolutely free from oil & fat. Also the amount of milk, which is animal product contains cholesterol, should be restricted. Thus, absolute vegetarian diet should be consumed which, is full of fibre and anti-oxidants.

## Stress Management

Stress being the most important cause of CHD, properly managing one's life is very important. The impact of stress can be reduced to a great extent if we can identify the cause of stress and find a remedy for it. We can atleast modify our reactions towards those causes, if it is not absolutely possible to eradicate them.

SAAOL enables one to identify their risk factors and accordingly modify them. This not only prevents heart attack, heart disease but also reverses heart disease.

# IMPORTANCE OF YOGA

## IN THE TREATMENT OF CHD

### Introduction

Yoga and Relaxation have been successfully used for the amelioration of high blood-pressure and coronary Heart disease over the past few decades. Recent researches have proved that this form of treatment not only reduces high blood-pressure but also reduces the serum Cholesterol levels, serum Triglyceride levels, serum free fatty acid, blood glucose, body weight and coronary artery disease. No form of medicine is as effective as yoga in the treatment of coronary heart disease. Unlike medical drugs, this form of therapy has no side effects. Yogic practice also improves physical fitness and helps to improve an individual's efficiency. Here, we are using a particular life-style enhancement intervention based on Preksha Yoga.

### Definition

Yoga is the philosophical doctrine developed in India in about 500 BC. Based on moral principles, meditational techniques and a special type of physical training called Hatha Yoga which involves control of posture and respiration... it is said to bring about the right interaction, combination, co-ordination of the mind and body.

**Saaol Recommends These Five Different Goups of Practices**

1. Heart Rejuvenating Exercises (HRE)
2. Asanas or Relaxing Postures

3. Pranayama or Breathing exercises
4. Kayotsarg or Relaxation
5. Meditation: Preksha Dhyaan
6. Moral Teaching & Anupreksha

**Training and Timings:**

Total duration of the daily practice of yoga should be about 40 to 60 minutes. However, meditation can be practiced for longer periods, if one desires. The best time to practice Yoga and Relaxation is early in the morning which is also very convenient for a regular practitioner or a professional who has to go to work everyday. Ideally, the stomach should be empty during the practice. Some of the optimum requirements other than these are loose and comfortably fitting clothes, quiet surroundings and an adequately ventilated room.

The training will consist of four separate sessions, each of 2 hours duration, where the patients along with their spouses will be taught all these procedures. They can however, consult the manual from time to time while they practice at home to verify any procedure.

**Rules and Regulations**

1. Regularity and punctuality in practice is essential.
2. The time fixed for practice should be maintained. Early morning hours are best suited for such types of practices because the bowels are clean and the stomach is empty. For some people evening hours are also suitable. At least 2 hours gap must be allowed between meals and practice.
3. If one needs a cup of coffee or tea or milk, it can be taken half an hour before the practice of asanas. The ideal goal of its practitioner is to stop tea and coffee completely.
4. **Place:** A clean and airy place without noise or disturbance is ideal for doing exercises and Asanas.

5. **Dress:** Comfortable, loose and a light dress is good for such practices.
6. **Sleep:** About 6 to 8 hours of sleep is required daily for an adult. If one goes to bed early, it will be possible to have a sound sleep and to get up early in the morning. Then and only then does it become possible to maintain the proper timing for Yoga practice.
7. **Rest:** While doing Asanas if one feels tired, he/ she should take rest. Never cross the limits of your capacity. Your capacity will increase slowly. After completion of the Asanas five minutes of Kayotsarg (muscular relaxation) is necessary. After that meditation can be practiced.

# HEART REJUVENATING EXERCISES

These few postural movements mentioned below are preparatory to beginning the next step i.e. Asanas. They are to be practised before beginning the Yogic training.

They are:-

I. For The Eyes
II. For The Neck
III. For The Ears
IV. For The Face
V. For The Shoulders
VI. For The Chest
VII. For The Waist
VIII. For The Thighs
IX. For The Knees
X. For The Ankle Joints
XI. For The Toes & Heels

## I. For The eyes

**A) Position:**

Stand at ease

**B) Movements:**

1. Keeping the head fixed look up and down a few times.

2. Then look to your right and left, and further rotate your eyeballs. Try to cover the maximum range.
3. Put your palms over both eyes after warming and blink a few times.

## II. For the Neck

**A) Position:**

Stand at ease.

**B) Movements:**

1. Rub the hands together vigorously for 10 counts. Rub the back position of the neck alternatively.
2. Repeat the same from the front side five times.
3. Bend your neck backward as far as possible and then touch your chin to the chest by bending forward. Repeat this procedure five times.
4. Turn your neck thoroughly from the left side, over the shoulders and vice-versa.
5. Bend your neck alternatively to both sides, try to touch the ears to the left and right shoulders alternately.
6. Rotate the neck starting with the chin, touching the chest with the eyes closed, turn to the right with eyes open, ears touching the shoulders and further through the back looking up and left ear touching the left shoulder and back to chin with eyes closed. Do it on the other side also (2 rounds).

## III. For the Ears

**A) Position:**

As above. Hold upper portion of both ears with thumb and index fingers.

**B) Movement:**

1. Pull up both ears.

2. Pull straight out the middle portion.
3. Pull down the lower lobes.
4. Cover both the ears completely with the palms, press and relax without taking away the hands to create vacuum in the ears.
5. Make fist with three fingers and thumb, leaving the index free. Now with the index fingers rub the front of the ears.
6. With the same fingers now rub the back side of the ears.

## IV. For The face

**A) Position:**

Stand at ease.

**B) Movements:**

1. Rub your face gently using both the palms.
2. Feel relaxed.

## V. For the Shoulders

**A) Position:**

Stand at ease.

**B) Movement:**

1. Keep your arms hanging straight down by your sides with fists closed. Raise the shoulders up, while inhaling and bring down while exhaling, without bending the elbows.
2. Rotate the shoulders from backward to forward keeping the arms relaxed and repeat it from forward to backward also (five time each).
3. Bend your arms, fingers and thumb together touching the shoulders. Inhale and rotate the arms from forward to backward and then from backward to forward.

## VI. For the Chest

**A) Position:**

1. Bend both arms inwards, bringing the palms over the chest, facing it, with middle fingers meeting at the middle of the sternum.

**B) Movement:**

1. Inhale and extend the left hand, exhale and bring the hand to its former position. Repeat the exercise with the right hand (five times each) and then do it with both the arms five times.
2. Keep the hands in front on the thighs. Inhale and raise the left arm touching the ear without bending, bring the arms down and exhale. Repeat it with right arm and then with both the arms five times.

## VII. For the Waist

**A) Position:**

1. Keep the feet apart as per the shoulder width. Arms should be hanging down by the sides of the body.

**B) Movement:**

1. Raise hands while inhaling, bend at the waist about 30° or more to the left while exhaling, bring the left hand near the knee, bend the neck to the left, drop the left hand also over the head, inhale and exhale for 3 times. Reverse the process and come to the normal posture. Repeat this on the right side (2 rounds).
2. Lock the fingers and raise hands.
   (a) Turn palm upwards towards the sky.
   (b) Bend at waist 30° or more to the left, arms straight with ears towards the left.
   (c) Return to the position (1).
   (d) Bring the arms down, repeat it to the right (2 rounds).

3. Keep the palms together.
   (a) Inhale and raise the hands upwards, arms straight touching the ears.
   (b) Exhale and bend 30° or more to the left. (Inhale & exhale for 5 times).
   (c) Return to position (a).
   (d) Bring the arms down, repeat it to the right.
4. (a) Inhale, raise the arms to shoulder level apart at chest width, keeping the palms facing each other.
   (b) Twist at the waist so that the right hand goes to the left shoulder and the left hand goes to the right hip. (Inhale and exhale 5 times).
   (c) Inhale and come to position (a).
   (d) Exhale and bring the hands down. Repeat the same on the right side (3 rounds).

## VIII. For the Thighs & Hips

**A) Position:**

1. Stand straight, keep the legs apart about 15 to 20 cm.

**B) Movement:**

1. Strike the buttocks with the heel; alternately.

## IX. For the Knees

**A) Position:**

1. Keep the above standing position.

**B) Movement:**

1. Let your left heel hit the hip; then stretch forward feeling the jerk at knee. Do it with right leg also. Repeat five times.
2. Place your hands on the waist keeping your thumbs in the front. Keep both feet 30 cms apart. Keep the body

straight and bend knees as low as possible, then, come up. Repeat this 5 times.

### X. For the Ankle Joints

Raise the left leg a little above the ground. Move the ankle upward and downward 5 times. Then rotate from the ankle clockwise and anti-clockwise. Repeat it with the right leg also.

### XI. For the Toes & Heels

Walk forwards on your toes, then walk backwards on your heels.

# THE YOGA EXERCISES

## STANDING POSTURES

### 1. TADASANA

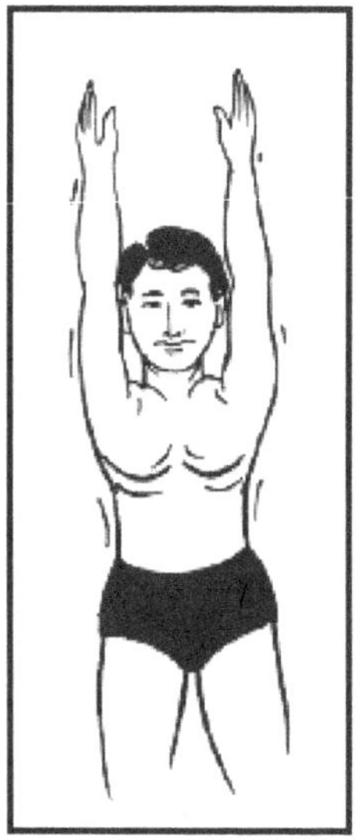

**Position** : Keep both heels and toes parallel and 10 cm apart; arms by the side.

**Movement :** Inhale. Raise the arms up, expanding the chest and abdomen slowly. Put the back side of the palms together, raise the body on the toes. Hold the posture looking at a point at eye-level. Keep the knees straight, bring the heels and arms down while exhaling as in the starting position.

**Caution::** Persons with slipped disc should not do this posture.

### 2. PADAHASTA ASANA

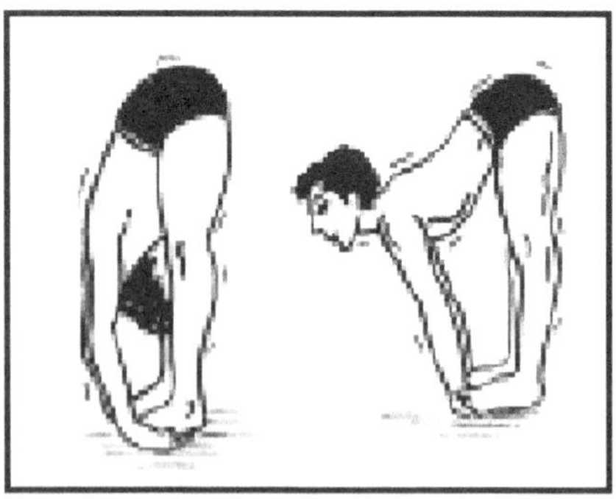

**Position** : Stand erect with both feet together.

**Movement** : Raise the arms, palms facing forwards over the head while inhaling. Exhale slowly while you bend forward, bring the palms down to hold the ankles and touch forehead to the knees.

Try to keep the knees and ankles straight. While you bend your body up to the level where you can bend easily keep in mind that the goal is to touch the forehead to the knees. Slowly raise your body while inhaling and taking the arms up exhale and bring the arms down.

**Caution :** Persons who have slipped disc (disc prolapse) should not do this asana.

## SITTING POSTURES

### 3. VAJRASANA

**Position :** Kneel down.

**Movement :** Assume kneeling position, heels open apart and toes together, soles upward. Sit on the soles, keeping the knees together. Inhale and exhale slowly and rhythmically.

### 4. SHASANKASANA

**Position :** Sit in Vajrasana. Put palms together on the knees, keeping both arms straight.

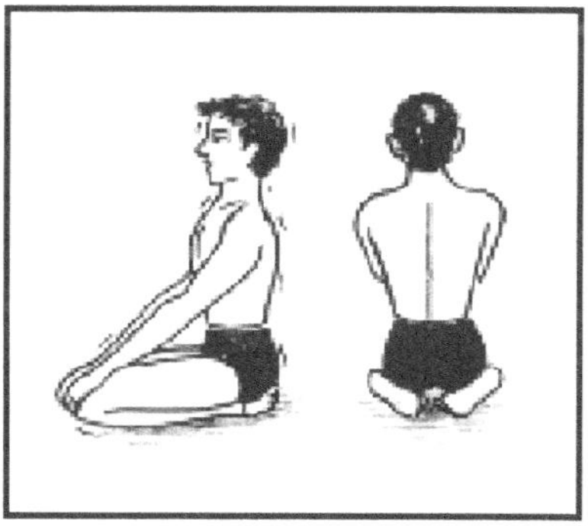

**Movement :** Inhale and raise the joined arms over the head. Arms should touch the ears. Exhale and bend forward touching the floor with the palms. Inhale Exhale and maintain this posture for five breaths. Inhale and raise the arms along with the head. Exhale and bring the hands down. Do it twice.

### 5. ARDHAMATSHYENDRASANA

**Position :** Sit on the floor with the legs stretched straight in front.

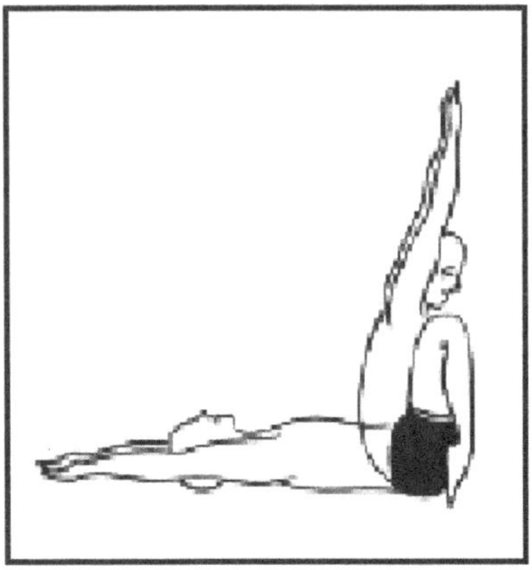

**Movement :** Raise the right leg a little and bend the left leg and let the heel touch the right hip.

Put the right leg and foot by the outer side of the left knee, sole on the floor. Bring the left armpit over the right knee, hold the right ankle with left hand. Exhale and stretch the right arm and swing back to touch the naval. Breathe evenly and maintain this posture for half a minute. Inhale and bring the right arm to the right side, exhale and free the left hand and legs. Repeat this on the other side.

## LYING DOWN ON CHEST POSTURES

### 6. SHALABHASANA

**Position 1** : Lie down on your chest with arms parallel to the body and chin on the ground.

**Movement 1 :** Inhale, turn the toes inward, heels high, exhale, make the body stiff and raise right leg up from the floor as Inhale and exhale and raise both the legs 15 cm high above the floor. Inhale and exhale for 5 times (inhale and bring the legs down and then exhale). high as you can. Hold, inhale and exhale for one minute.

1. Inhale and bring down the leg on the floor slowly and exhale.
2. Repeat with the other leg.
3. Now repeat with both the legs.

## LYING ON THE BACK ASANAS

### 7 UTTANPADASANA

**Position :** Lie down on the back keeping the fingers locked

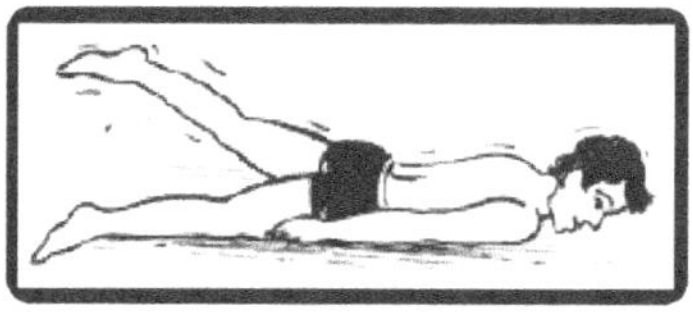

together, under your neck, elbows on the ground. Keep the feet 15 cm apart.

**Movement :** Inhale and exhale and raise both legs 15cm high above the floor. Inhale and exhale for 5 times (inhale and bring the legs down and then exhale.)

**Position 2 :** Keep the legs 25 cm apart

**Movement :** Heels out, toes in, and raise the legs 15 cm above the floor. Inhale and exhale for 5 times. While inhaling, bring the legs down and exhale and relax. ;

**Position 3 :** Keep legs 45 cm apart

**Movement :** Do the same set of movements. Relax

## 8. MERUDANDASANA

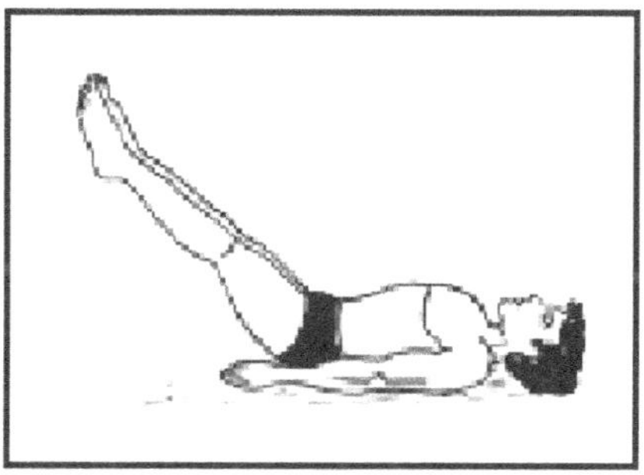

Lie on the back with the arms stretched at right angles to the trunk. Lift the left heel and put it on the right foot in the space between the big toe and the second toe, thus, keeping the feet straight one above the other. Now stretch and rotate the upper part of the body (head and neck) towards the left and the lower parts (waist, thighs and feet) towards the right while you inhale. The left toe should now touch the ground and the arms and shoulders remain in the same position as before. Now come back to the original position while you exhale. Now repeat the same on the other side.

Repeat the whole process after changing the leg position (Right heel over the left foot).

## PRANAYAMA

### (NADI-SHODHAN PRANAYAMA)

Sit in a comfortable posture and breathe normally. Close your right nostril with your thumb and inhale slowly through the left nostril. When the inhalation is complete, close the left nostril also and hold your breath for 2-3 seconds. Now lift the thumb from the right nostril and slowly exhale keeping the left nostril closed. Repeat the process by inhaling through the left nostril and exhaling through the right nostril. This is one cycle of Nadi-shodan pranayama. Repeat this for 10 cycles.

# KAYOTSARGA

## (Relaxation with self awareness)

This is an important practice of Preksha Dhyaan. The literary meaning is "*To drop the body*". 'Kaya' means "*Body*", and 'Utsarga' means "*to drop or abandon*". In practice it is conscious suspension of all the gross movements of the body. The result is relaxation of the muscles and reduction of metabolic activities. This physical condition helps in relieving mental tension. Physically it is more restful than sleep and is the most harmless and direct antidote to psychosomatic maladies resulting from stress and anxiety. Progressively all the muscles are relaxed.

### The Technique

This exercise can be done in any posture such as sitting, standing or lying down. When we practice meditation, it is essential that the practice be done while sitting. When we want to be free from tension, this is done in the lying down posture.

### The Pledge

In the standing position the pledge is to be recited. "I want to be free from my physical, mental and emotional tensions, for that I practice KAYOTSARGA. I pledge that I will maintain awareness throughout the practice". Lock the hands and give tension to the whole body by stretching it upward raising the body on the toes and feel the tension in every muscle.

**Step - 1 :** Sit or lie down keeping the spine and neck straight but without stiffness, eyes softly closed. Relax all the muscles of the body and let them become limp.

**Step - 2 :** Focus your attention on each part of the body one by one. Allow each part to relax by auto-suggestion and feel that they have become relaxed.

**Step - 3 :** For deep relaxation of body and mind start with the big toe of the right foot; suggest muscles and nerves to relax, feel them relaxed and pass on to the other parts of the right leg-toes, sole, heel, ankle, calf muscles, knee, thigh, and buttock. In the same way also relax the left leg.

**Step - 4 :** Relax the trunk from the hip joint to the neck, starting with the back and front of the lower abdomen, upper abdomen, ribs, front and back, chest muscles, collar bone and the neck muscles. Then relax the right hand starting with tips of fingers upto the shoulder then the left hand from the tips of the fingers to the shoulder joint.

**Step - 5 :** Relax the upper part of the body from neck to head and throat, chin, jaws, lips, tongue, mouth, cheeks, nose, eyes, ears, temples, forehead, and the scalp of the head.

**Step - 6 :** Feel and experience that the whole body is completely relaxed. When the body and mind is relaxed, maintain this condition for a few minutes.

**Step - 7 :** Perceive the whole body and feel it physically, mentally and emotionally relaxed. If there is any tension in any part, relax it again, and once again feel the whole body totally relaxed. Maintain this posture for a few minutes.

**Step - 8 :** To finish Kayotsarga, the body has to be charged with energy part by part, inhaling fully into each part. Start with the upper part of the head, face and neck, the middle part of the trunk, the right hand, then the left hand, the right leg and the left leg. The whole body! Inhale and turn to the left side placing the elbows below the neck. Slowly sit up. Take two or three full breaths.

# THE CONCEPT OF CALORIES IN FOOD

Body is a machine that keeps on working through out the day. For all the activities that we perform in our daily routine like eating, sitting, cooking, driving, walking, talking, swimming and running our body needs energy. This energy comes from the food in the form of calories.This calorie is similar to petrol as a fuel for car i.e.fuel for our body is calories.

**What is Calorie?**

As we measure money in rupees, weight in kilograms, energy is measured in calories. Any work we do we need calories. If I talk for a minute, I will need about two calories. If I run, I need about 10 calories in a minute. For any work we need calories. Even when we sleep the body has to keep on beating the heart and breathing and these will need about half a calorie every minute.

**How do we know that how much fuel is required by our body?**

Answer is requirement of fuel depends upon the **Physical Activity** of the person.Physical Activity is directly related to the calorie requirement.

Let us make a list of our daily activities like reading,eating, sitting, driving,talking.... for all these work our body spends very less calories. Such type of work is called Sedentary Work.So, how many calories are required by a sedentary worker. The answer is 1600 calories per day. But labourers and heavy workers require more calories as their physiological need is high.

**What is Your Calorie Spending?**

In a day of normal activities for most of common people (those not engaged in physical labour) require about 1600 calories in a day. A labourer may require 3000 calories. If you don't do any work and only sleep throughout the day and night, you will probably require about 800 calories per day. I am giving you a chart about how many calories are usually requires when one does usual activities.

Body requires minimum calories at the time of rest i.e.0.5 cal/min and at the time of running maximum calories are required i.e.10-12 cal/min.A table for approximate energy expenditure is given below to roughly assess how many calories we use doing our daily regular activities:

| Work Approximate Per Minute | Calories |
|---|---|
| Sleep | 0.6 calories |
| Reading | 1.4 calories |
| Eating | 1.8 calories |
| Converse | 1.8 calories |
| Writing | 1.9 calories |
| Standing | 2.2 calories |
| Driving a car | 2.1 calories |
| Slow walking | 3 to 4 calories |
| Casual walking | 4 to 5 calories |
| Fast walking | 6 to 8 calories |
| Jogging | 7 to 9 calories |
| Running | 10 to 12 calories |

Now, this is all about the expenditure. For expenditure we need income i.e.money. Income for our body comes from food that we eat.

**What we eat as a food?**

We eat Salads, Chapati, Rice, Vegetables...As for example:

In South India people eat-

Idli, Dosa, Sambhar, Uttapam, Coconut chutney...

In North India we eat-

Chapati, Dal, Rice, Vegetables, Parantha...

In America we eat

Sandwiches, Burger...

In Italy we eat

Pizzas,Pasta ...

Can you count the total number of dishes? There will be hundreds and thousands of dishes in the whole world. Can you count the calories of all the dishes? No, its difficult. To make it easy our medical science has divided all the dishes into seven groups. All the dishes in the world can be put into two categories and seven groups.

| CATEGORY I | CATEGORY II |
|---|---|
| CARBOHYDRATES | VITAMINS |
| PROTEIN | MINERALS |
| FATS | FIBRE |
| | WATER |

The difference in the category I gives calories and category II does not give calories for example if we drink a glass of water it will give us zero calories.On the other hand :

- 1gram of CARBOHYDRATE give 4 cal
- 1gram of PROTEIN give 4 cal
- 1gram of FATS give 9cal

**Components of Diet :**

FATS such as all types of oils like Saffola/ Dhara/ Groundnut/ Olive oil/ Soyabeen oil/ Ghee/ Butter/ Cream. Fats are the concentrated source of energy providing 9cal/gm and are made of fatty acids of different proportion.

PROTEINS such as animal food like Milk/ Meat/ Fish/ Eggs and plants food such as Legumes and Cereals are rich source of proteins. Animal protein is good in quality as they provide all the amino acids in right proportions but they are rich in cholesterol.A combination of Cereals, Millets, Pulses provide better quality of proteins. Proteins perform a wide range of functions and also provide energy 4 cal/gm.

Now,whatever foods are left all are considered as CARBOHYDRATES such as Rice/Chapati/ Potatoes/ Glucose/ Sugar. All cereals like Rice,Wheat, Bajra, Fruits, Orange, Apple, banana, mango, cheeku,papaya all come in carbohydrates. Let us see where all can carbohydrates be found.

For exanple have you eaten Glucose how it tastes - sweet and what about Chapati how it tastes - is it sweet? No, it is not sweet. It gives a bland taste.So, all the foods which taste sweet are simple carbohydrates and which are not sweet to taste are called as complex carbohydrates

Most of our body cells utilize Glucose as a major source of energy. Carbohydrates are the main source of glucose in the body and our food mainly consists of carbohydrates (such as Chapatti, Rice, Ragi, Kowar, all vegetables etc) which help to maintain normal blood glucose levels. Thus a Diabetes patient must select the kind of carbohydrates which will constantly supply the blood with glucose, but will not suddenly increase the blood glucose levels. Diabetics should avoid simple Carbohydrates and instead consume complex Carbohydrates. How we test which food is simple Carbohydrate or which food is complex Carbohydrate.we are going to test all the foods through a laboratory.Practically it is not possible.God has given all of us a laboratory to test the food that is tongue.Taste a little amount of food if it tastes sweet it is simple carbohydrate and the food which do not taste sweet is complex Carbohydrate. Hence diabetics should avoid all the food that tastes sweet.

If the brain wants sweet taste we can make use of artificial sweetners like Sweetex, Equal, Aspartame etc.

Now one has to use knowledge and common sense in selecting the fruits. Fruits which taste sweet when put into mouth should not be taken by diabetics as they contain plenty of simple carbohydrates. Sweet fruits thus increase blood sugar.

Take for example the case of 'papaya' There are always two kinds available in the market. 'Disco papaya' and 'Desi papaya'. Disco papaya is very sweet while Desi papaya is non-sweet. Disco papaya is mostly red or reddish and sweet, so it should be avoided. Desi papaya are yellowish and are not sweet as they have more complex carbohydrates and can be consumed in good amounts.

Similarly in almost every fruit there are two varieties, sweet and non- sweet. So diabetics should take the non-sweet variety of fruits, like, Pomegranate, Watermelon, Apple, Orange, Mausami, Guava, Papaya.

Four fruits that need to be strictly avoided by diabetics are:- Mango, Banana, Grapes and Cheeku as they are always sweet.

At last what is more important for diabetic is balanced diet. All the components of diet should be adequately present in ones meal to meet the daily requirements.

# WHAT IS BALANCED DIET?

The diet containing all the essential nutrients like carbohydrates, protein, fats, vitamins, minerals, fibre, water in optimum quantities and in appropriate proportions to meet the requirement of the body.

So, Calorie break up is:

| | | | |
|---|---|---|---|
| Carbohydrate | - | 70% - | 1120 calories (280gm) |
| Protein | - | 20% - | 320 calories (80gm) |
| Fat | - | 10% - | 160 calories (18gm) |

We don't have to take fats at all so, where this 10% fats comes from? This 10% comes from all the pulses, cereals and vegetables. All the food we eat contains some amount of invisible fat (fat present as an integral component of plant and animal foods such as cereals, legumes, spices) in it. That is we do not have to take visible fat(Fats and oils that can be used directly or in cooking).

Somebody asks a question, "When we have to eat this 1600 Calories? before breakfast or after breakfast? It is to be consumed in the whole day. How many times we eat the food. Four times

| | | |
|---|---|---|
| BREAKFAST | 30% | 480 cal |
| LUNCH | 30% | 480 cal |
| TEA | 10% | 160 cal |
| DINNER | 30% | 480 cal |

After dinner what we do? Nothing, we only go to sleep and in sleeping how much calories are spent i.e. only 0.5 cal/minute. Therefore, we reduce the calories by 5% and it is to be added to lunch. Now the calories break up to 1600 calories is

| | | |
|---|---|---|
| BREAKFAST | 30% | 480 cal |
| LUNCH | 35% | 560 cal |
| TEA | 10% | 160 cal |
| DINNER | 25% | 400 cal |

# ZERO OIL CONCEPT

The commonest form of lifestyle, which people have in this modern era, is sedentary lifestyle. Very few are involved in regular physical activity. Most of us have a lifestyle which has minimal of physical work, no exercise and bad dietary habits i.e. sedentary lifestyle.

Now, it is known to all that fat forms blockages in the arteries (tubes which carry blood) like coronary arteries. These fats are called cholesterol and triglycerides. They get deposited in layers over a period of years. When these blockages become significant the tubes (arteries) get choked leading to a disease called coronary artery disease (angina, heart attack).

In the past 50 years cholesterol (an animal fat) was considered as the only constituent of the blockages. It was only in the last one decade or so that Triglyceride (a plant fat) has been found to be equally responsible for creating blockages. Triglyceride is the chemical name, known to the common man as "Cooking Oil". The oil manufacturing companies exploited the naivety of the people, misled them to believe that oils are harmless by promoting their sales with captions like "Cholesterol Free" or "Zero Cholesterol Oil". Well, it is true that oil does not have Cholesterol because it is made from plant seeds whereas cholesterol comes from animal products (meat, milk & their products). The lay man started buying these oils. What they failed to realize was that these oils are also hundred percent fats because they are Triglycerides and Triglycerides are equally harmful. Oils also have high calories content (each gram gives nine calories) that can lead to obesity, diabetes and high blood pressure. It is best to minimize the fat content in our food (optimum requirement of fat by the body is 10% of the total calories).

This can be easily obtained from all the food items, as every food contains oil known as invisible fat or hidden fat. This means that all the visible sources of fat (i.e. cooking oil) should be completely cut down. Now, this would raise a query: How to prepare delicious food without oil?

**Zero oil means no visible oil (cooking oil). The body requirement for fat is met by invisible oil (naturally present in food items).**

What if the food is prepared without oil? Will the taste be there? If you think rationally the answer would be yes. The taste comes from the spices (Masalas). Oil itself does not add taste. It is our mindset, which was trained to believe all these years, which says that taste comes from oil. But when we ask to remove the oil, the masalas get removed automatically. This happens because the housewife does not know how to put the spices, when no oil appears in the frying pan. This prompted SAAOL to develop the concept of "Zero Oil". By "Zero Oil" we mean cooking without using a single drop of oil. SAAOL cooks the spices and food in water and since the spices are there the color, taste and flavor remain intact.

SAAOL also realizes that the mindset of people finds it difficult to accept water as the cooking media. So we have named water, when used as cooking media - ***"SAAOL Oil"***. By introducing the zero oil concept in your cooking there will be no risk of taking in cholesterol & triglycerides. This can also be helpful in reducing weight, since the high calorie gain from fat is removed.

We can now aptly say that SAAOL Oil contains no fat, no cholesterol, is 100% mineral and good for health.

# QUICK DEFINITIONS

**Metabolism** is the biological process by which energy is extracted from the foods consumed, producing carbon dioxide and water as by-products for elimination. Metabolism involves catabolic and anabolic activity. The catabolic function controls digestion, disassembling food into forms the body can use for energy, while the anabolic function produces substances for cell growth and repair.

**Calorie,** is a measure of the energy-producing potential contained in food. In practical terms, the number of calories in a particular food tells you how much fuel you're getting from eating it.

**Glucose**, a type of sugar, is the main fuel used by the brain. After a meal is eaten, the pancreas produces insulin to enable sugar to be metabolized. If you are eating a lot of carbohydrates, your body will become assustomed to producing a lot of insulin and over time, you may experience insulin resistance. The result is your body may store the carbohydrates as fat rather than be made available as fuel that can be burned off by your body as energy.

**Glucagon** is secreted by your pancreas and helps to unlock the body's fat stroes to be burned as fuel. If too much insulin is present in the bloodstream, such as following a steady diet of carbohydrates, glucagon is blocked. Fat is not freed up to be used and the dieter often craves more carbohydrates as he or she may feel lethargic, unable to gain access to the energy locked in the body's fat stores.

**Hypoglycemia**, or low-blood sugar, is a condition often associated with dibetes. Symptoms include anxiety, weakness, sweating, rapid heart rate, dizziness, headache, irritability, and poor or double vision, among others.These symptoms commonly occur in mid-afternoon, when most people experience a slight drip in blood sugar (Glucose) levels.

**Diabetes mellitus** is a degenerative illness that centers around the hormone insulin and the pancreas. In type I diabetes, also called juvenile diabetes, the pancreas is unable to manufacture insulin. Type II diabetes, or noninsulin dependent adult-onset diabetes, develops in middle-age. Here, the pancreas produces insulin, but the body's cells do not respond to it and can't absorb the glucose from food. As blood glucose levels continue to rise, the pancreas released more insulin to deal with the excess blood sugar. The result is both a state of low blood sugar and too much insulin (Hyperinsulinism)

**Omega-3** and **omega-6** oils are the two principle types of essential fatty acids, which are unsaturated fats required in the diet. A balance of these oils in the diet is required for good health. The primary omega-3 oil is alphalinotenic acid (ALA) found in Flaxseed, Canola, Pumpkin, Walnut, and Soyabean, Fish oils, such as Salmon, Cod, and Mackerel, contain the other important omega-3 oils, DHA (Docosahexaenoic acid)and EPA (Elcos-apentaenoic acid). Linoleic acid is the main omega-6 oil, gammalinolenic acid (GLA), is found in evening primrose, black currant, and borage oils.

An **Antioxidant** (meaning "against oxidation") is a natural biochemical substance that protects living cells against damage from harmful free radicals. Antioxidants work against the process of oxidation-the robbing of electrons from substances. If unblocked or left uncontrolled, oxidation can lead to cellular aging, degeneration, arthritis, heart disease, cancer, and other illnesses. Antioxidants in the body act readily with oxygen breakdown products and free radicals, neutralize them before they can damage the body. Antioxidant nutrients include vitamins A.C, and E, beta carotene, selenium, coenzyme Q10, pycnogenol (Grape seed extract), L-giutathione, superoxide dismutase, and bioflavonoids,. Plant antioxidants include Ginkgo biloba and garlic. When Antioxidants are taken in combination, the effect is stronger than when they are used indivdually.

# FATS AND OILS

**Q1. Why do you recommend zero oil food?**

**Ans.** Heart diseases have (coronary artery disease) become very common in the present world. There are various risk factors leading to this disease but the commonest one is the food habits and the lifestyle. In Indian culture food plays a vital role. Festivals, ceremonies etc. are lavished with variety of foods specially made of oil and ghee. Such foods contribute to high calories. Overweight is yet another problem faced due to such foods. When the intake of fat foods increases the fat content in our body increases and as we know fat takes longer time to get digested so it stores in our body, which leads to obesity. When there is excess of fat in the blood it settles in the arteries and create blockages. So, when there is so much fat in the body we do not recommend oil in the food and insist on zero oil food so that the fat deposited in the arteries as blockages meets the requirement of the fat in the body.

**Q2. How does oil affect our heart?**

**Ans.** All oils are 100% fats and the major content of these oils are Triglycerides. In heart disease the problem is blockage or deposition of fats inside the tubes supplying blood to the heart. Amongst the two types of fats, that make the deposit one is Cholesterol and other is Triglyceride. When excess amount of oil is taken in our food it increases our blood levels of Triglycerides. When the blood level of Triglycerides exceeds a particular level (above 130mg/dl) more blockages are formed. Thus all the oils are bad for the heart and push up the chances of blockage.

The possibility becomes more in the modern mechanized society- when we are exercising less and less. Most of our time we spend sitting and doing low-grade physical activity (watching TV, working on computers, driving cars, talking on telephones) – which do not help in digesting the oil that we take in most of our food.

**Q3. What are Triglycerides?**

**Ans.** Triglycerides are nothing but fats. More than ninety nine percent of the fats that we consume are Triglycerides. Less than one percent that is left out is Cholesterol. All the fats of plant origin (example: Sunflower oil, Olive oils, Palm oil, Groundnut oil, Mustard oil, Coconut oil, Vanaspati) are nothing but Ttriglycerides. Fats of animal origin have some minute amount of Cholesterol- but rest of the fats are Triglycerides.

Scientifically speaking, Triglycerides are made up of one glycerol molecule and three molecules of fatty acids. Triglycerides also can give energy or calories to the body. One gram of Triglyceride will give 9 calories to the body. The usual blood level of Triglyceride is 40-160 mg/100 ml of blood. If this level is towards the upper end of the range or above 160 mg/100ml they will start depositing inside the arteries of the body – especially the coronary tubes or arteries. This is why those who eat a lot of fat or Triglycerides or oil are prone to Heart disease and ultimately get heart attacks.

SAAOL recommends heart patients to keep the blood level of Triglycerides at least below 130mg/100ml.

**Q4. What are mono unsaturated oils?**

**Ans.** Triglycerides are made of glycerol and three fatty acids. These fatty acid chains contain carbon and hydrogen atoms. Each carbon is attached to two hydrogen atoms. When one hydrogen atom is removed from fatty acid chain it forms mono unsaturated oil. These oils are equally harmful and create blockages like Cholesterol. Example: olive oil.

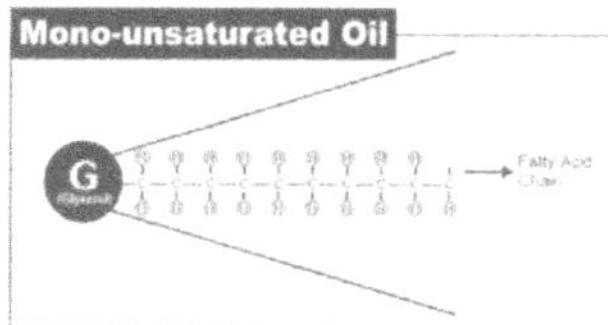


## Q5. What are Poly -unsaturated oils?

**Ans.** When in fatty acid chain one or more than one-hydrogen atoms are removed it forms polyunsaturated oil. Consumption of these oils also leads to heart problems because they are Triglycerides and are known for blockages in the arteries. Example: Sunflower oil, Safflower oil.

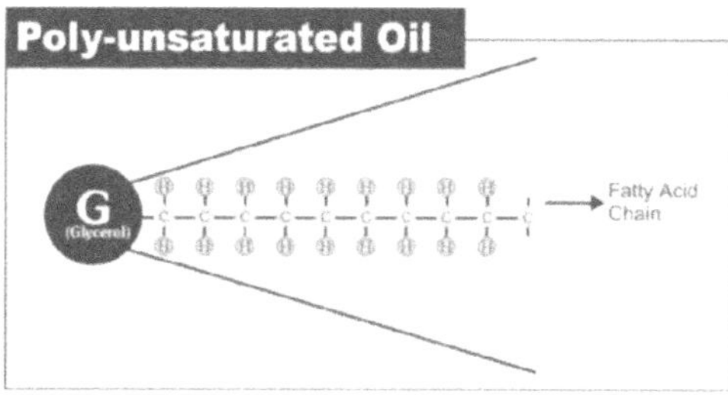


## Q6. What are Saturated oils?

**Ans.** When in fatty acid chain all the carbon atoms are attached to two hydrogen atoms and there is no carbon atom left without hydrogen attachment it forms saturated oils. Oils can be saturated with the process of hydrogenation in which hydrogen is passed through the oils and it hardens. Example: Vanaspati, Dalda, Ghee.

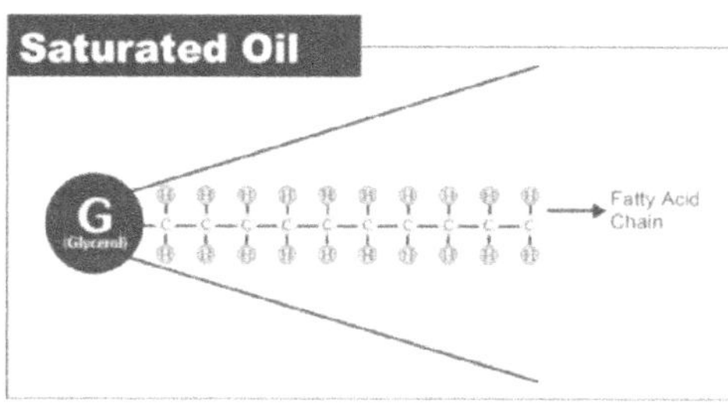


## Q7. Can I take Ghee?

**Ans.** It is common belief in India that consuming fat or oil in form of Ghee gives strength to the body and also provides nutrition. Oil is taken by us in two forms either directly i.e. adding Ghee or oil in the curries, which is also called visible oil or it is obtained from the plants and animal product, which we consume. This is natural oil present in them and is called invisible oil.

No, you cannot take Ghee because it is a saturated fat, which is rich in cholesterol. Cholesterol is known for creating blockages. So, we completely avoid Ghee in our patient's diet.

**Q8. Can I take Fish oil?**

**Ans.** It is a general belief that fish oil is good for heart patients, because it contains more omega-3 fatty acid compared to omega 6 fats but here we would like to inform you that this oil is obtained from animal source (Fish). Any oil from animal source will have high Cholesterol and Cholesterol is a primal cause of blockages. So, we do not recommend fish oil. In fact you can take cereals and pulses, which are plant sources of omega-3 fatty acids and are not harmful for your heart.

**Q9. Can I take Margarine?**

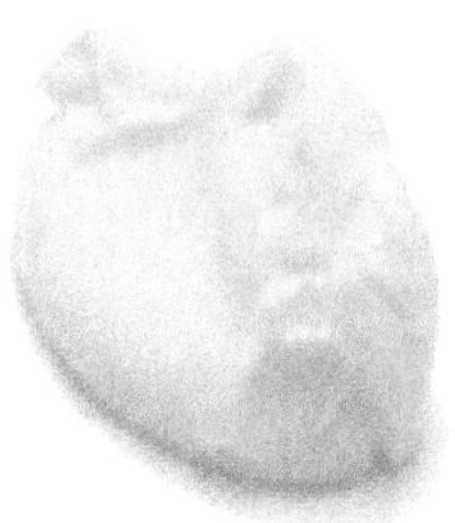

**Ans.** If you leave a cube of Margarine sitting out for years moulds, insects or rodents will not touch it. It would appear that only humans are foolish enough to eat it. Margarine is 78% saturated fat and known to be a nonfood item. Adding hydrogen atom to a fat molecule makes it saturated fat. This process is called hydrogenation. Margarine is partially hydrogenated and various metal catalysts are used for this process. It not only causes heart problems but also leads to various types of cancers. So, here we would not recommend Margarine to heart patients at all.

**Q10. Olive oil is said to be good for the heart. Is it true?**

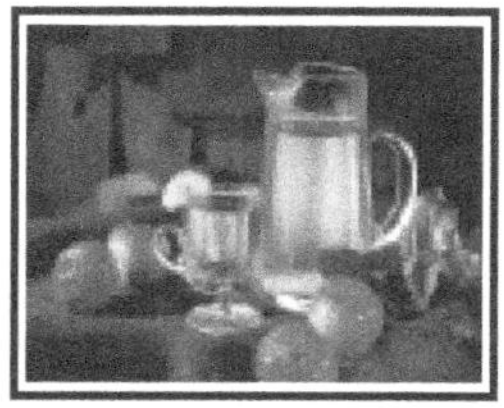

**Ans.** Many patients/people consume these expensive oils thinking they are good for heart, which is not true. Olive oils are high in mono unsaturated fatty acids (98.5%), which unlike saturated fats do not adversely affect blood cholesterol levels but they are rich in Triglycerides. Triglycerides are another known cause for blockages so, heart patients should avoid olive oil.

**Q.11. Can we apply Oil on our body surface?**

**Ans.** Yes, you can apply oil. Oil free diet can cause dryness on your skin so to avoid this dryness oil can be applied. Applying oil on the body surface does not affect adversely i.e. it does not get absorbed in such a way that it can affect your heart.

**Q.12 Many companies sell oils with various labels, e.g. "Cholesterol Free", "Heart Friendly" etc. Are they true?**

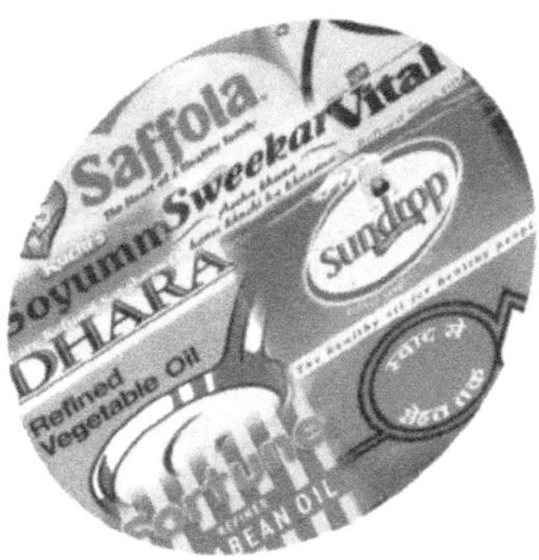


**Ans.** Oil companies promote their oil by labeling various slogans like, "Heart Friendly Oil", "Cholesterol Free", "Helps Reduce Cholesterol level etc. All these labels are untrue. The fact is that cholesterol is present only in animal products. And since all these oil come from plant products, there is no question of cholesterol being present in them. In fact they contain Triglycerides, which are equally harmful and forms blockages in the heart.

**Q13. What is "SAAOL Oil"?**

**Ans.** Water is called SAAOL oil, which is recommended by SAAOL. As we know water does not contain Triglycerides and

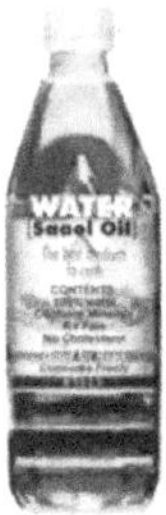

cholesterol, so it cannot lead to blockages. It also enhances natural flavor of masalas and one can use it to any limit. Water as a cooking medium is safe and healthy. The masalas are roasted first then purees are added and when it sticks little water is added. SAAOL has already developed more than 1000 tasty recipes using this water (SAAOL oil).

**Q14. Why do we know more about Cholesterol as a major causative agent of Heart disease then Triglycerides?**

**Ans.** In the present medical world Cholesterol and Triglycerides have proved themselves to be the culprit for heart related problems. We know more about Cholesterol as a major causative agent of heart diseases because it was discovered about more then five decades ago that Cholesterol creates blockages whereas it is recently proven that Triglycerides are also major causative agent of blockages.

**Q15. Can we take some oil in case we are looking only for prevention and do not want reversal?**

**Ans.** Yes, you can take oil in case of prevention and are not looking for reversal. For reversal Saaol recommend 18gm of oil from invisible sources. In case of prevention you can take 18 gm from invisible sources and 18 gm from visible sources. If exceeded this recommendation you may suffer from heart problems.

**Q16. Should children go on a 10% fat diet?**

**Ans.** No, children should not go on 10% fat diet till 18years of age. It is so because it is their growth phase in which, there requirement for fat specially for Cholesterol is more as it is used in development of nerves in nervous system.After 18 years if they want they can follow 10% fat diet.

**Q17. How to Cook without Oil?**

**Ans.** In every day cooking it is a pattern to add oil and then masalas. We believe that without oil food cannot be cooked but it is possible with saaol way of cooking.The saaol way of cooking is

- Heat a kadhai (preferable non-stick pan).
- Dry roast the jeera (cumin seeds) until it crackles and turns brown.
- Add ground onion in the kadhai (non-stick pan) and keep roasting it. When it starts sticking upon the hot surface, add small amount of water and keep stirring.
- Add ginger and garlic paste (according to your taste/wish).
- Roast the onion, ginger, garlic till it turns to brown. (Note: Do not add more water at a time as it gives the food – a boiled taste.
- Then add tomato paste in the kadhai and roast it with little amount of water. Roast till the water bubbles start forming.
- Add the turmeric powder and cook for some time (as turmeric takes time in cooking).
- Finally add all the masalas/spices like salt, red chilli powder and coriander powder according to the taste.
- Now, the zero oil masala is ready.
- If you want to make vegetable – add vegetables.
- If you wish to cook dal – add boiled dal or soaked dal. Cook as required.
- Add garam masala (A combination of cloves, mace, nutmeg, black cardamom, red chillies).
- Garnish it with finely chopped coriander

**Q18. Does dietary cholesterol affect blood cholesterol levels?**

**Ans.** Dietary cholesterol does affect your cholesterol level. It is true that saturated fat will affect it even more but the amount of cholesterol in your diet is an important factor in your blood cholesterol level. It is shown that even a single meal that is high in fat and cholesterol may cause your arteries to constrict and your blood to clot faster. The amount of blockage in your arteries is only one of several factors that affects your heart.

**Q19. What is visible or invisible oil? what all foods contain invisible oil?**

**Ans** Oils or fat can be classified into two categories: visible and invisible oil. Visible oils are which we see packed in cartons and bottles example sunflower oil, mustard oil etc.

Invisible oils are those which can not be seen but is present in the food items naturally.

The food items containing invisible oil are :

| Name of the food stuff | gm per 100gms |
|---|---|
| Barley | 1.3 |
| Maize | 0.9 |
| Rice | 0.5 |
| Wheat | 1.5 |
| Suji | 0.8 |
| Urad | 1.4 |
| Matar (Dry) | 1.1 |
| Razma | 1.3 |
| Chaulai | 0.7 |
| Bathua | 0.4 |
| Pudina | 0.6 |
| Potato | 0.1 |
| Pumpkin | 0.1 |
| Apple | 0.5 |
| Guava | 0.3 |
| Musk Melon | 0.1 |

**Q20. What are the best ways to lower your Triglycerides?**

**Ans** The best ways to lower your Triglycerides are the following:

Reduce oil intake because they are nothing but Triglycerides and also reduce your intake of sugar and other simple carbohydrates, including white flour, white rice, and alcohol, which your body converts to sugar. These simple carbohydrates are absorbed quickly, causing your blood glucose (sugar) level to rise quickly. In response to this, your pancreas secretes insulin to lower your blood sugar to a normal range, which is good. However, insulin also accelerates the conversion of calories into Triglycerides.

Complex Carbohydrates, sometimes called "whole foods," include fruits, vegetables, grains, and beans in their natural forms, such as whole wheat flour and brown rice. These foods are rich in fiber. Fiber slows the absorption of food, so you don't get a rapid rise in blood glucose and excessive insulin production. Also, you get a more constant source of energy throughout the day.

# CEREALS

### Q21. Can I take Dhokla?

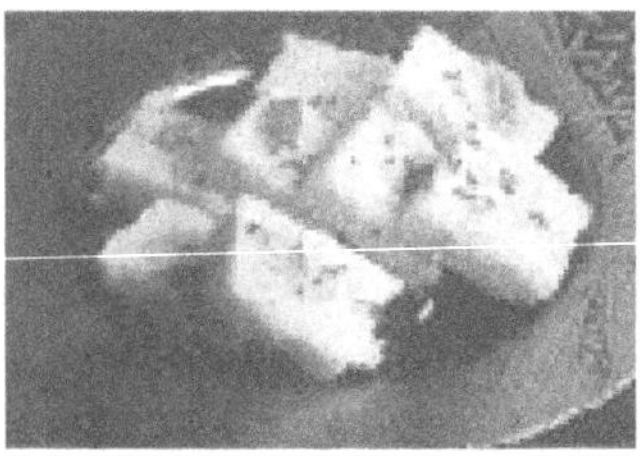

**Ans.** Dhokla is a Gujrati dish. It is made of besan and curds. It is a fermented product, which is good for digestion. After steaming, it is cut into small pieces then it is sauted with mustard seeds and chillies. In case of heart patients dhokla can be eaten if curds is made up of skimmed milk and seasoning should not be done with oil.

### Q22. Can I eat Naan?

**Ans.** Naan is a flat teardrop shaped yeast leavened bread, baked on the hot side of the tandoori oven. It is madeup of maida, which is refined wheat flour and low in fiber content. Being low in fiber content it is to be taken moderately by heart patients.

### Q23. Can I eat Bread?

**Ans.** Yes, you can eat bread but before eating, you should know that there are two types of bread one is white and other is brown bread. White bread is made up of maida and has low fiber content. Whereas brown is

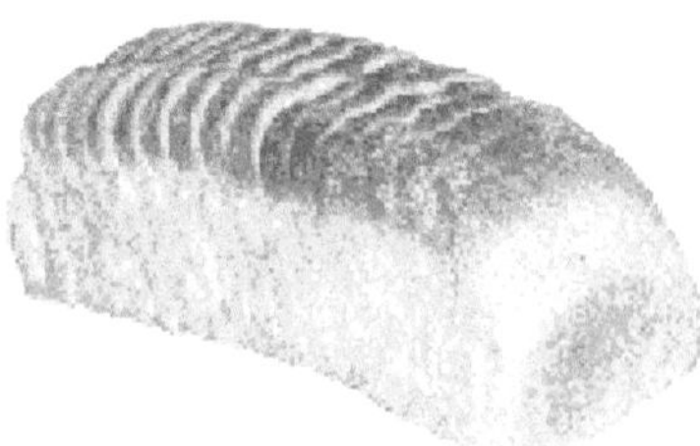

made up of whole wheat, its fiber content is high. Making vegetable sandwich, vegetable like cucumber, onion, tomato, cabbage etc can be used, can increase the fiber content of white bread.Remember bread has lot of calories so should be taken moderately by overweight.

**Q24. Can I eat Macaroni?**

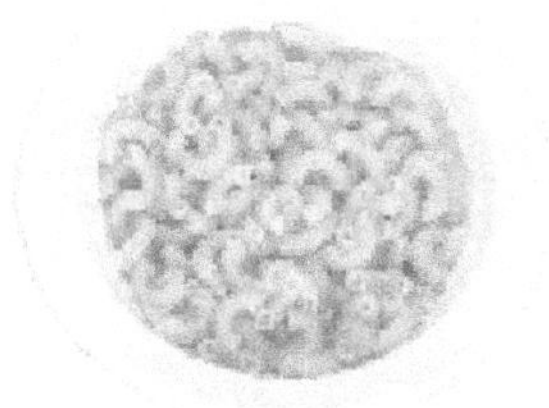

**Ans.** Macaroni is an Italian dish. It can be eaten moderately by heart patients because it is made up of refined flour. It is made by forcing stiff dough through metal plates under pressure . To cook, boil macaroni then add tomato sauce, vegetable and other flavoring agents. Adding more of vegetables can increase fiber content of macaroni.

**Q25. Can I eat Noodles?**

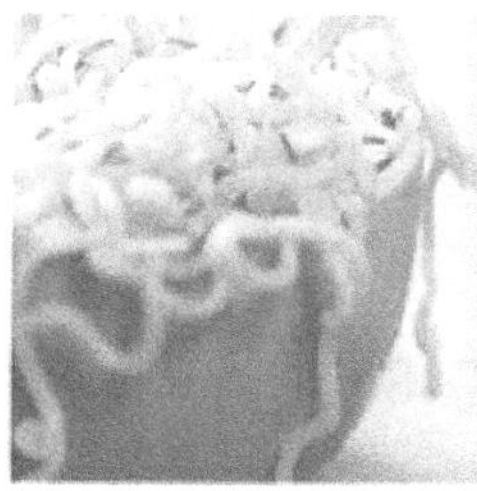

**Ans.** Noodles and all other pasta products can be eaten moderately by heart patients They are all made up of maida which is refined and contains negligible amount of fiber. One can eat macaroni and other pastas without restriction by mixing whole lot of green vegetables like onion, carrots, capsicum, peas etc.

**Q26. What is Wheat Bran (Choker)?**

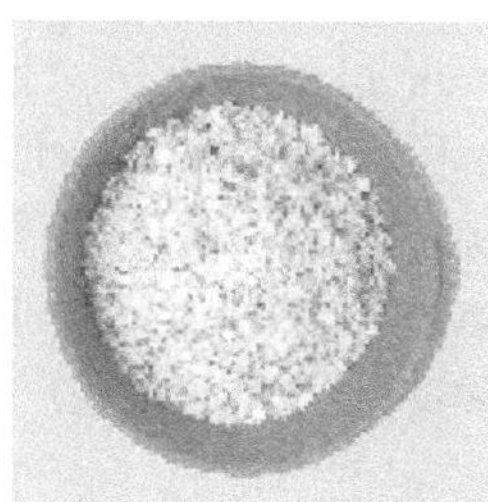

**Ans.** Wheat bran or choker is nothing but husk of wheat. It is a complete fiber. It contains nearly all the cellulose of the entire grain. It has various beneficial effects. It is an essential requisite for removal of constipation as "laxative effects of bran are much superior to those of fruits and green vegetable for the reason that cellulose of latter is more readily or easily broken down by bacteria while passing through the intestine.

**Q27. Why Oatmeal is suggested to Heart patient?**

**Ans.** Oat is jayee, which grows plenty in Rajasthan. Now, oat and oatmeal has become popular all over the world. Oatmeal is good for heart patients. Oat bran is a vital source of fiber, which helps to control the levels of cholesterol in the body. It contains oat germ, which is more nutritious than wheat bran. A couple of bowl of oat bran and three bowls of oatmeal a day can depress cholesterol 10 percent or more depending on individual responses. Oats helps to stabilize blood sugar, Oestrogenic and antioxidant activity. They also contain psychoactive compound that may combat nicotine cravings and have antidepressant powers but high doses can cause gas or abdominal bloating. These effects are negligible.

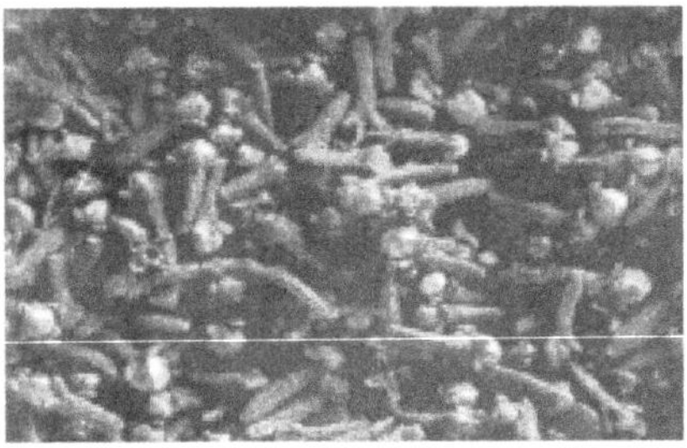

**Q28. Can I take Corn/Makai?**

**Ans.** Yes, you can take corn. Corn in India is same as maize in the west. In nutritive value whole corn slightly exceeds wheat. It is sweet, nutritious and palatable. Corn has anticancer activity. The fiber content of corn is high which helps in binding cholesterol and lowering its level in blood. Corn can be consumed as corn flakes, roti, dalia or as salad (after boiling)

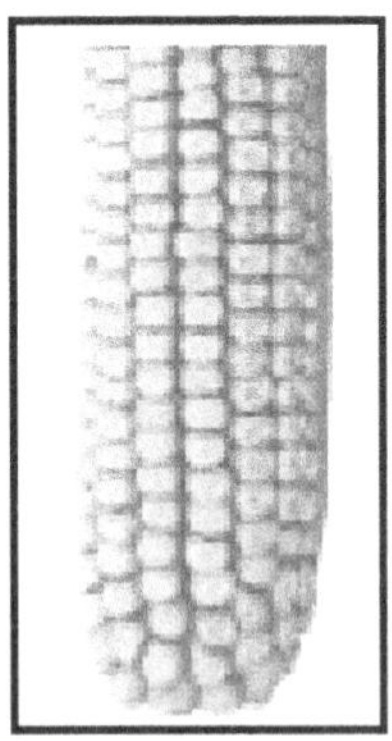

**Q29. What is khakra?**

**Ans.** Khakra is a gujrati dish. It is prepared by making dough of gram flour and other spices like salt, chilli, garlic-onion paste. Roll into thin rotis. Roast them on slow flame by pressing them with cloth. Finally it will become in the form of papad. There are different verities of khakra- methi khakra, gram flour khakra, onion khakra, and tomato khakra.

**Q30. What is Brown Bread?**

**Ans.** Brown bread is nothing but bread, which is made of whole-wheat flour. It contains good amount of B-complex vitamins and is rich in fibre. Fibre is a good cholesterol-lowering agent. So it can be taken freely by heart patients.

**Q31. What is White Bread?**

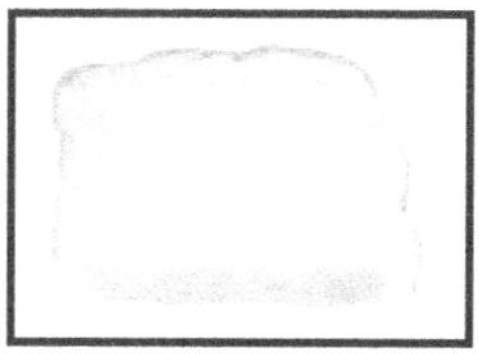

**Ans.** White bread is made with flour milled from the inner part of wheat grain after the husk has been removed. It also contains water and yeast along with various additives, preservatives and emulsifiers.

**Q32. Why Brown Bread is considered good than white bread?**

**Ans.** Brown bread is considered good than white bread because brown bread has more fibre than white bread. It is even good for diabetics. It is a weight reducing snack.

**Q33. Can I eat Cakes?**

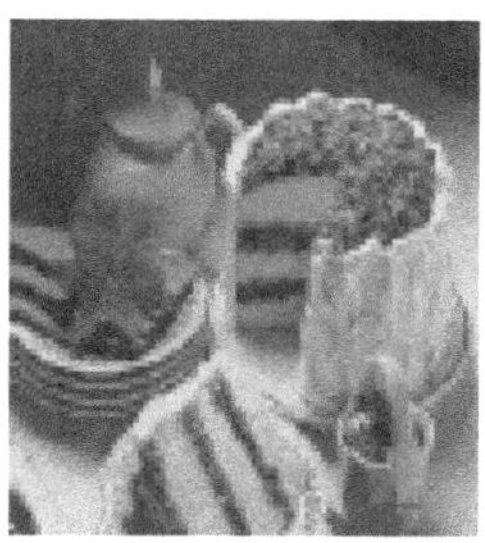

**Ans.** No, you cannot eat cakes. Cakes are bakery item, which are made with maida, sugar, salt, eggs, milk, and cream. These cakes are high in calories and have lot of saturated fat. They also have high dietary cholesterol, when made with lot of eggs, butter or cream. All these ingredients are linked with heart diseases. Some cakes claim to be healthy as they are made of fruits or carrots but they tend to have high sugar and fat content. So, to avoid further complications it is better to avoid cakes.

**Q34. How the calories of Chappati can be reduced?**

**Ans.** The calories of chapatti can be reduced in the following way- By adding green leafy vegetables. Soya flour Besan Vegetable stuffing Wheat bran Chapatti by mixture of two or three flours i.e. missi roti.

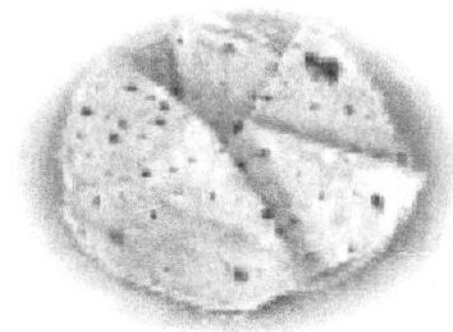

**Q35. How one can decrease the calories of the Rice?**

**Ans.** One can decrease the calorie of the rice in the following ways-

- By removing the starch
- By adding green leafy vegetables.
- By consuming brown rice which has more fiber than white rice.

**Q36. Why whole Wheat Dalia is good for heart?**

**Ans.** Whole wheat dalia is good for heart patients as it is rich in fiber. Fiber is cellulose which is obtained from whole grain and help in reducing cholesterol levels. Whole wheat dalia is nothing but broken wheat which is used in number of snacks like broken wheat porridge, vegetable dalia, dalia-upma etc.

**Q37. Can I eat Podi with Rice?**

**Ans.** Yes, You can eat podi with rice. It is very delicious and nutritious combination. Podi is a south Indian recipe made up of dal, which is roasted, and other masalas like chilli powder, dhania powder, salt, curry leaves are added. Then it is ground to coarse powder. If you add water to it, it becomes dal chutney.

**Q38. Can I take Germinated Wheat?**

**Ans.** Yes, you can take Germinated Wheat. Germinated; wheat is very nutritious. It is rich in B-complex, vitamin C, and minerals. It also helps in easy digestion of food. This Germinated Wheat is also used for making baby foods.

**Q39. What is wheat Grass?**

**Ans.** Wheat Grass is nothing but the small wheat saplings, which comes out after germination. These small wheat plants are rich source of vitamins and minerals. They also have laxative properties and help in various stomach disorders. It improves oxygenation. This is the reason for using Wheat Grass juice to improve circulatory system.

**Q40. Can I eat Missi roti? Why usually combination of Cereals and Pulses is suggested?**

**Ans.** Yes you can eat Missi roti. Missi roti is combination of various flours. This combination of flour makes it a complete food. If we add soyabean flour to wheat flour we get nutrition of both cereals and pulses. A part from that this combination helps in reduction of glucose and cholesterol levels of blood because it has high fibre content.

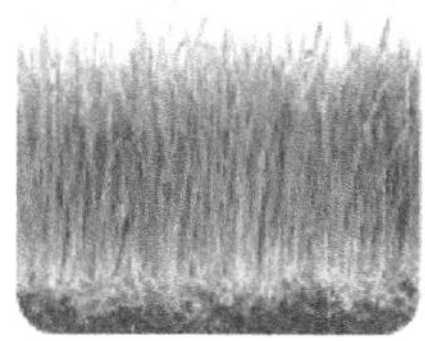

**Q41. Why Soybean is suggested for heart patients?**

**Ans.** Soyabean – "the miracle golden bean" may be considered as the king of pulses. It is rich source of protein. It is proven that soyabean protein reduces cholesterol levels. It also has high fiber content which reduces blood sugar levels. When the cholesterol levels are low there are less chances of blockages and further heart disease.

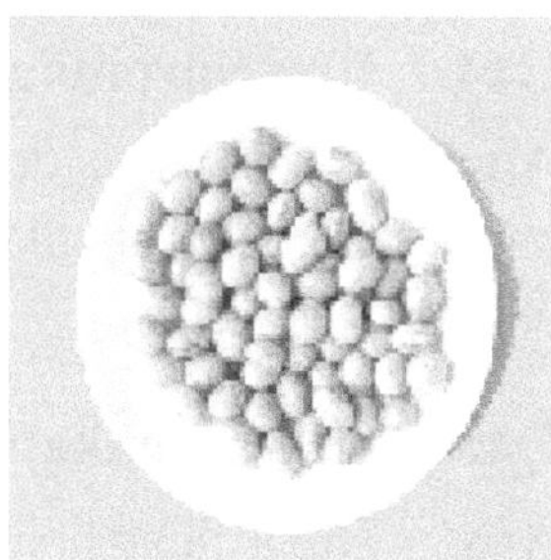

**Q42. What is Tofu?**

**Ans.** As cheese is to milk tofu is to soyabean. It is also known as "Cheese of Asia". Soft creamy colored Tofu is made by grinding cooked soya beans to produce milk that is then solidified with a mineral coagulant (calcium sulphate). Tofu is high in protein, very low in saturated fats and cholesterol free , a 100g serving of steamed tofu contains 73 calories. Tofu is naturally bland and can therefore be used in both sweet and savoury dishes.

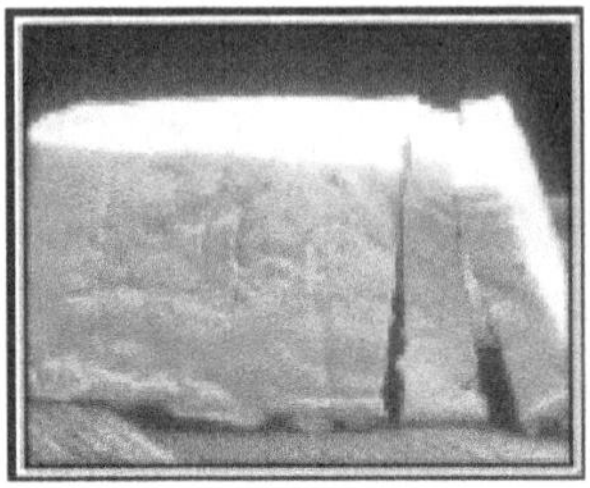

Benefits of tofu are:

- High in protein.
- Low in saturated fats.
- Good source of calcium and a useful source of vitamin E.
- May help to protect against some forms of cancer and heart disease.

**Q43. Can we consume unlimited amount of Soyabean?**

**Ans.** No, one should not consume as much soyabean as one wants. Because soyabean is very high in protein and consumption of high amount of protein will effect kidney functioning. It also has high amount of fat which can lead to heart problems. It should only be used after processing (meal maker, Tofu etc).

**Q44. How Sprouts are good for heart?**

**Ans.** Sprouts are good for the heart as it is rich in fiber and natural antioxidants like vitamin C and E. Sprouts also help in reducing the weight.

**Q45. How to make Sprouts?**

**Ans.** Dip a clean neat piece of cloth in water, rinse out extra water. Thereafter where grains/pulses should be put into the moistened cloth and then knotted or bound with some thread. It should be ensured that cloth does not get dried up, so occasionally keep on moistening. After 36-48 hours the grains will sprout, being ready to eat, preferably in the morning or when required.

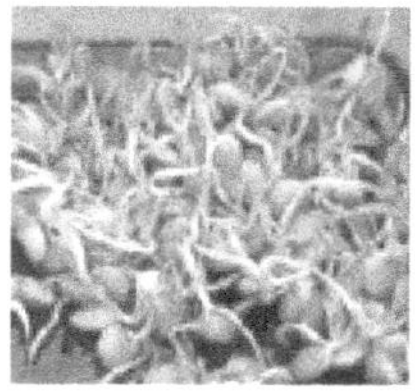

**Q46. What is meant by Cereals and Pulses with Husk?**

**Ans.** Cereals and pulses with husk mean cereals and pulses with covers. The fiber of the cereals and pulses is present in the covers. Having cereals and pulses with covers means an increment of fiber in the diet. It will also reduce the calories of cereals and pulses.

**Q47. What is the difference between good Carbohydrate and bad Carbohydrate?**

**Ans** Good Carbohydrate are not processed and contain a fair amount of fibre (i.e. whole grain bread, oatmeal and whole grain cereals, legumes, veggies, fruits) etc.

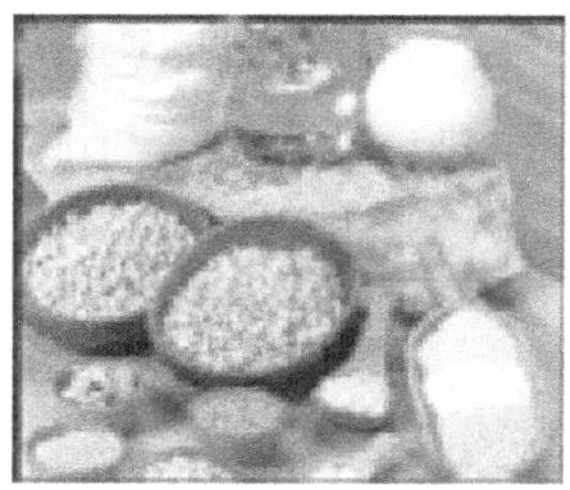

Bad Carbohydrate are refined or processed (i.e. white bread, white pasta, soda, sugary foods including ice-cream). It is recommended that you select whole grain carbohydrate over sugary or processed carbohydrate, however, you can incorporate small portions of refined carbohydrate into your diet on occasion and still lose weight. The key will be small portion.

# MILK & MILK PRODUCTS

**Q48. Why Milk is restricted for heart patients?**

**Ans.** Milk is an animal product and contains about 4-6% of fat. Moreover being an animal product it has cholesterol in it. As we know in coronary heart diseases main culprit are cholesterol and Triglycerides. Which are supplied abundantly by milk. Milk contains 11mg/100ml of cholesterol. Earlier people used to consume more milk and their hard working lifestyle use to burn their extra calories. In present times people have sedentary lifestyle and are not able to burn their calories so milk is no help instead it leads to problems.

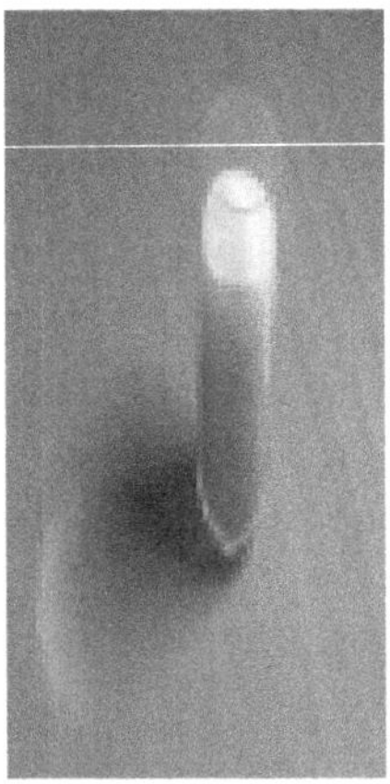

In spite of high content of fat milk is a good source of calcium, potassium, protein and vitamins. It is liked all over the country and abroad. There are two recommended way of fat removal –

1. Milk should be boiled and allowed to thaw and cream on top of it is removed and then it is refrigerated. Again it is heated and the cream is removed. With this removal very little amount of cholesterol (5mg/100ml) is left. SAAOL recommends 200ml of such milk in a whole day.
2. There are many dairies and milk corporations, which are selling skimmed milk.

**Q49. Can I take Chenna/Paneer?**

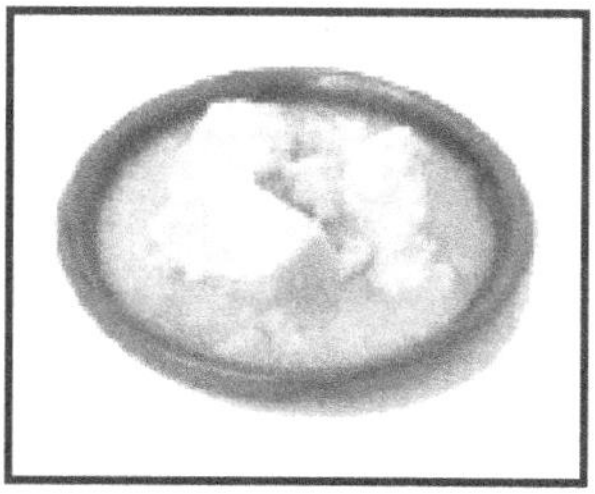

**Ans.** Chenna is a milk product. It is commonly known as Paneer. It is made out of milk by curdling it and removing the whey water. Chenna or Paneer has 25% fat in it. If 500ml of milk is curdled we get 100gm of paneer. This shows how concentrated paneer is. It is used in various delicacies mostly in north India. Sweets like sandesh, rasogolla etc. are made out of it. Whereas heart patients are concerned they cannot take chenna made out of whole milk. SAAOL recommends chenna made out of skimmed milk, which has very less fat around 0.1%. Instead of milk chenna tofu is a best substitute. It is made of soya milk, which is known for its cholesterol lowering property.

**Q50. What is Toned Milk?**

**Ans.** Toned milk is that milk, in which the fat content of the milk is reduced to a very less amount. Whole milk has around 4% fat, in toning of milk it is reduced to 3%. Toning can also be done at home. In this process milk is boiled and refrigerated then the scum or malai is removed. SAAOL recommends 200ml of milk of this kind.

**Q51. What is double Toned Milk?**

**Ans.** Double toned milk is that milk in which the toning is done mechanically in the dairy. In this process the fat content is reduced drastically .The double toned milk contains 0.5% fats. Heart patients can use this milk under SAAOL recommendation of 200ml/day.

**Q52. What is Skimmed Milk?**

**Ans.** Skimmed is another mechanical process in which the fat content of whole milk is reduced to around 0.1%. This milk is very good for those who wish to loose weight and also for heart patient.200ml of skimmed milk can be taken per day.

### Q53. Can I take Condensed Milk?

**Ans.** Condensed milk is a concentrated form of milk. In which the liquid percentage of water is very less. In this milk the nutrients are dense. It is good for those who are willing to put - on weight and is not heart patient. But heart patient cannot take this milk because along with other nutrient like proteins, calcium, etc. fat content is dense. If this concentrated form of milk is taken it can lead further to blockages. So heart patient cannot take this milk.

### Q54. What is Slim Milk?

**Ans.** Slim milk is nothing but another name of skim milk. To make people aware and conscious of their health, the dairy corporation e.g. (Mother dairy, Nestle) has released this milk in tetra packs. Earlier milk powder was available but people wanted natural form (liquid form). This milk is easy to consume and good for health.

### Q55. Can I take Butter?

**Ans** No, butter cannot be taken by obese and heart patients.

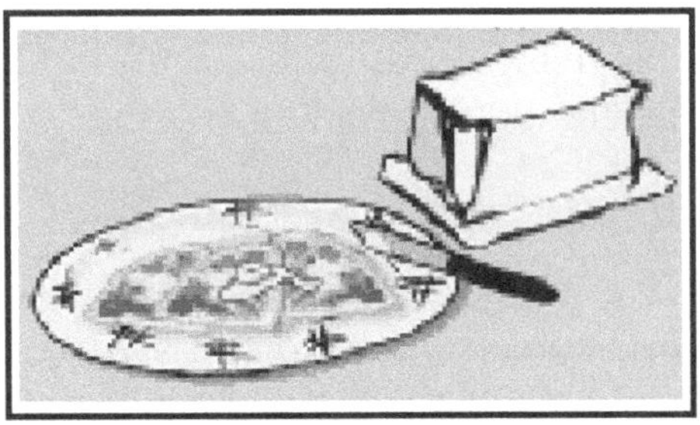

Butter is nothing but cent percent fat. It formed by churning cream, which is fat in it self. Butter is a milk product and contains cholesterol in it. We also know cholesterol is a known causative agent for blockage and heart diseases. In earlier times people use to eat butter as a energy source. They use to burn calories by hard working but in present sedentary life style it is not possible. And it is surely impossible for a heart patient to burn these extra calories. SAAOL recommends only 18 gm of fat that too from invisible sources. So it is not possible for a heart patient to take butter at all.

**Q56. Can heart patient take low fat Butter?**

**Ans** There is no such butter, which has low fat in it. It is a skill to market it. In America they sell this kind of butter with many things added to it, which makes available fats low. But it has fat in it. Which is equally harmful to heart patients. So they cannot be taken this is so called low fat butter.

**Q57. Can I take Curd?**

**Ans** Yes, you can take curd. Curd should be made out of skimmed milk or toned milk. SAAOL recommends 200ml of milk in a day. So you can make curd out of it.

**Q58. Can I take Shrikhand or Yogurt?**

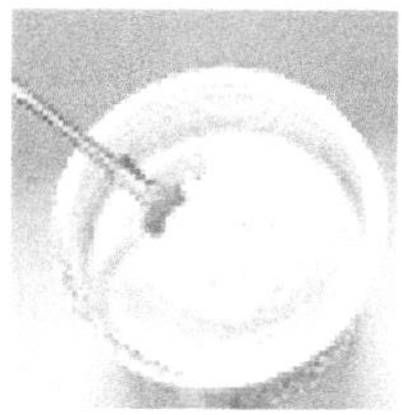

**Ans** There is a difference between shrikhand/condense curd and yogurt, shrikhand is made of mixed strains of lactobacillus whereas yogurt is made of specific strain. Yes, you can eat Shrikhand or Yogurt if it is made up of skimmed milk.

**Q59. What is Yogurt? Can heart patients take Yogurt?**

**Ans** Yogurt is pasteurized-homogenized milk to which bacteria culture is added. Yogurt is a useful source of calcium and phosphorus it also contains vitamins like $B_{2,}$ $B_{12}$ which help to replace valuable bacteria in the gut and boost the immune system. High fiber yogurts, with added soluble fiber, are being promoted for their cholesterol lowering properties. So it is advisable to take skim milk yogurt for heart patients.

**Q60. Can I take Buttermilk?**

**Ans** Yes, you can take Buttermilk. Buttermilk is a milk product and is made by churning curds to liquid consistency. Majority of the cream in form of butter is removed from it during the process. So there is no harm in taking diluted butter milk from 200ml of toned or skim milk.

**Q61. Can I drink Lassi?**

**Ans** In India especially in Punjab Lassi is famous. It is a milk product made by churning thick curds with cream in it. Cream is rich source of fat and fat is not good for heart patients as it leads to blockages. Heart patient can take lassi only if cream is removed from it and it should be made out of skim or toned milk. It is moderately allowed.

**Q62. We don't have easy access to toned milk, so, can we take milk from our local milkman?**

**Ans** Yes you can take milk from your local milkman. It is good in one way because they are clever enough to remove cream from it before selling milk. If your milkman is honest enough you can remove the cream by boiling the milk, cooling it and refrigerating it for six hours and then removing cream for it. Milk should be boiled again and again cream should be removed. This process should be repeated for two times at least.

**Q63. If Non – Veg is banned and milk intake is restricted, how one should make up for protein deficiency?**

**Ans** If Non – Veg is banned and milk intake is restricted one can easily make up for protein deficiency by eating lot of vegetarian foods like green leafy vegetables e.g. Spinach, Methi, and Bathua etc. Pulses like combination of beans, Moong Dal, Bengal gram dal etc. milk products, which are made of skimmed milk e.g. curds, paneer etc. Whole grains like Jowar, Whole wheat, rice etc. Other things like sprouts Mushrooms, Egg white etc.

**Q64. If milk intake is restricted than how to make up for the calcium requirement?**

**Ans** If milk intake is restricted than calcium requirement can be met easily. There are many calcium rich foods. Ragi is the richest source of calcium. Green leafy vegetable like spinach **(73mg/100gm)**, chaulai **(200mg/100gm)**, carrot leaves

**(340mg/100gm)**, and cauliflower leaves **(626mg/100gm)**, colocasia leaves (Arbi ke patte) **(460mg/100gm)**, drumstick leaves **(440mg/100gm)**, turnip leaves (Shalgam ke patte) **(710mg/100gm)**etc. Fruits like amla **(50mg/100gm)**, cherry **(24mg/100gm)**, guavas **(50mg/100gm)**, and lemon **(70mg/100gm)**. Other vegetables like beans **(80mg/100gm)**, drumstick **(30mg/100gm)**, jackfruit **(30mg/100gm)**, karonda **(21mg/100gm)**, kamal kakdi **(405mg/100gm)**, water chest nut (Singhada) **(20mg/100gm)**.

### Q65. Why Milk is not a good way to get Calcium?

**Ans** The problem with drinking milk as a source of calcium is that you are more likely to excrete calcium, because milk is high in animal protein as well as high in calcium. When you eat a lot of animal protein, your kidneys excrete more calcium along with the animal protein, so you end up "chasing your tail." It is found that who eat high animal protein diets tend to have a high incidence of osteoporosis. On the other hand, who eat more plant-based diets lower in animal protein have much lower rates of osteoporosis. Osteoporosis is not just due to an insufficient intake of calcium. It results from an imbalance between calcium intake and excretion.

### Q.66. Is there any Milk which does not have Cholesterol?

**Ans.** Both cholesterol and saturated fat in your diet may increase blood levels of cholesterol and increase the formation of plaque (blockages) in arteries. As you know, the reversal diet is designed for people with diagnosed heart disease, and it is more restricted than the prevention diet, which allows for a greater intake of fat and cholesterol. Yes, there is a non fat milk. Soy milk has no cholesterol, and soy products actually lowers your blood cholesterol levels. Soy is also rich in a number of substances that may have anti-cancer properties, paticularly with respect to prostrate cancer and breast cancer.

## MEAT AND EGG

### Q67. Can I eat Fish?

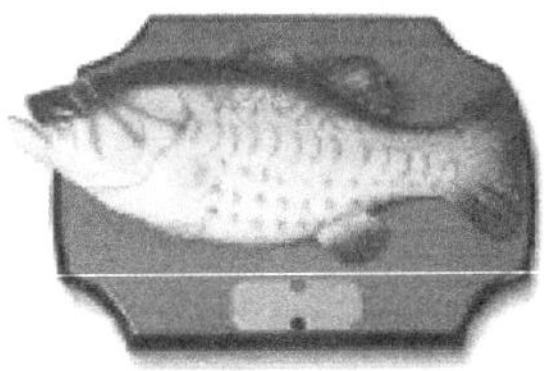

**Ans** No, you cannot eat fish. Fish is one of the most valuable sources of proteins and fats, besides having the advantage of being easily digested, compared with meat.

Two groups of fishes are commonly categorized as fat and lean. Fat fish include Herrings, Kippers, Salmon and Sardines, lean fish or white include Haddock, Sole and Turbot.

All fish is rich in minerals, vitamins and in protein, which are easily digested.

Even then fishes are not allowed for eating as they are very rich in cholesterol and cholesterol is an important risk factor for heart disease.

### Q68. Can I take Red Meat?

**Ans** No, you cannot eat red meat. Red meat includes the flesh of all mammals- such as deer, rabbit, and the edible portions of livestock such as cows, pigs, calves, or sheep. Most of the fat is unsaturated and relatively less is saturated. But both the fat increases cholesterol and Triglyceride levels in blood and thus leading to heart disease or heart attack.

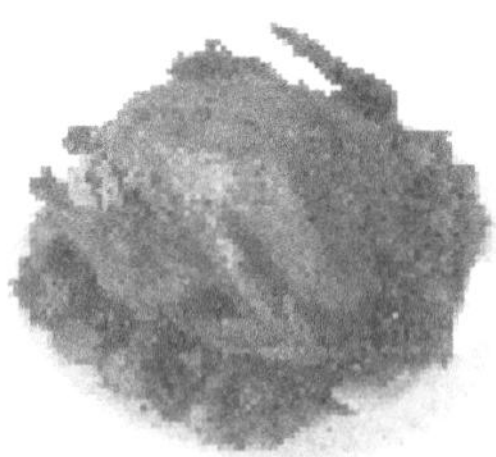

**Q69. Why Eskimos who are Meat and Fish eaters have low rate of heart disease?**

**Ans** Eskimos live in the toughest terrain and have to be phsically very active to survive. It is estimated that an average Eskimo spends 5000 calories/day. Whatever fat they eat - in fact are broken by them during the severe physical exercises.

This is why most of the labourers do not get heart problem even if they consume fat and meat.

**Q70. Can I take lean Meat/Chicken?**

**Ans** No, you cannot take lean Meat/Chicken. Lean meat is meat of chickens; farm-reared ducks, turkeys and geese and is also known as poultry. They all contain protein that builds and repair body tissue, plenty of vitamins for a healthy nervous system and some zinc. Most of the fat in poultry is unsaturated and relatively less is saturated. But both the fat increases cholesterol and Triglyceride levels in blood and thus leading to heart disease or heart attack.

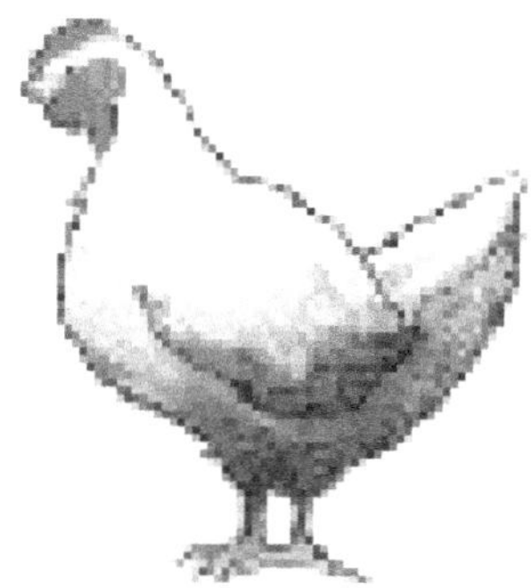

**Q71. Can I take Beef Meat?**

**Ans** No, you cannot take Beef. Beef is the meat of cows and is most commonly used but not so much in India. Though it contains a wide range of nutrients including valuable minerals, particularly iron and zinc.

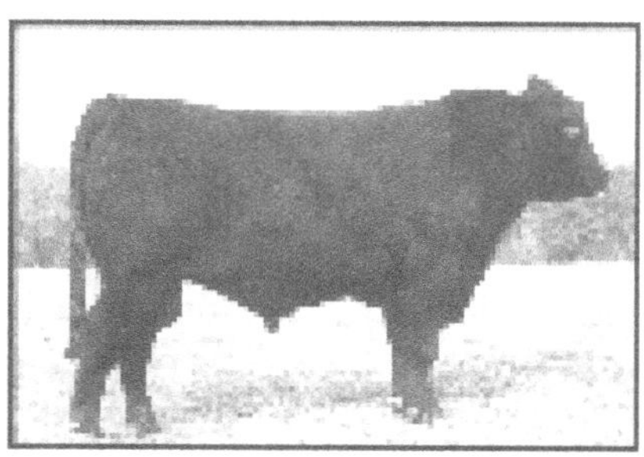

But high intake are linked to cancer of colon and too much beef meat can contribute to heart disease as it is rich in cholesterol and high blood levels of cholesterol is an important cause of heart disease.

**Q72. Can I eat Pork?**

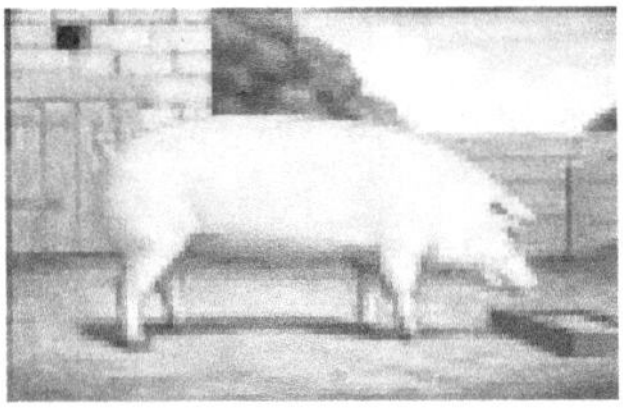

**Ans** No, you cannot eat pork. The flesh of the pig or swine is known as pork and is generally recognized as being less wholesome and less digestible than most other meats. Pork is high in saturated fat and excessive intakes of which are associated with high levels of cholesterol, hardening of the arteries and heart disease.

**Q73. Can Heart patients take Egg?**

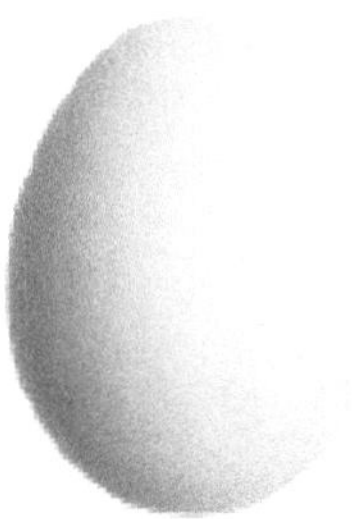

**Ans** An egg is designed by nature to provide protein, vitamins and minerals. Egg supplies a multiplicity of vitamins and minerals. In particular they are an excellent source of vitamin B12 and a convenient source of protein and rich in vitamins and minerals.

A large egg contains 6-8g of protein and 5-7g of fat of which less than 2g. is saturated. A single egg yolk provides 448 mg of cholesterol. In fact, the greater health concern is not dietary cholesterol but excessive blood cholesterol manufactured by the liver from saturated fats. The relatively high cholesterol content of eggs is only of concern to people who already have raised blood cholesterol level. So heart patients cannot take egg yolk but they can take egg white which is rich in albumen and it is more easily digested than egg yolk.

# LEAFY VEGETABLES

## Q74. Can I take Betel Leaves?

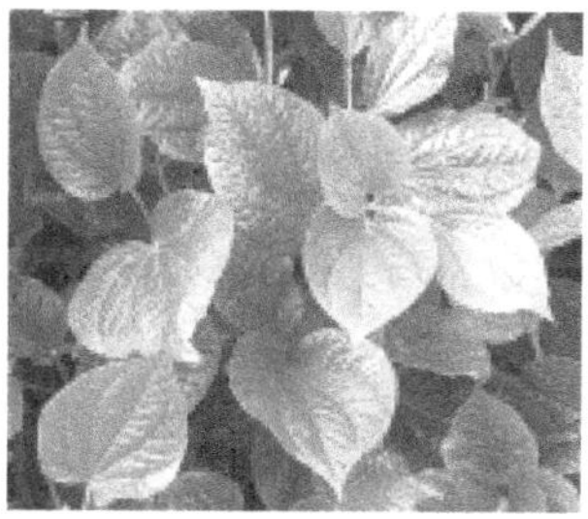

**Ans** Yes you can take betel leaves but it should be taken moderately. Betel leaves are commonly called as pan. Betel leaves have many desirable properties. They contain good amount of calcium, vitamin A, iron, manganese and also vitamin C. They have a medicinal and therapeutic effect. Betel leaves are chewed for their flavour and have refreshing digestive, calmative and stimulating properties.

## Q75. Why leafy Vegetables like Spinach are preferred?

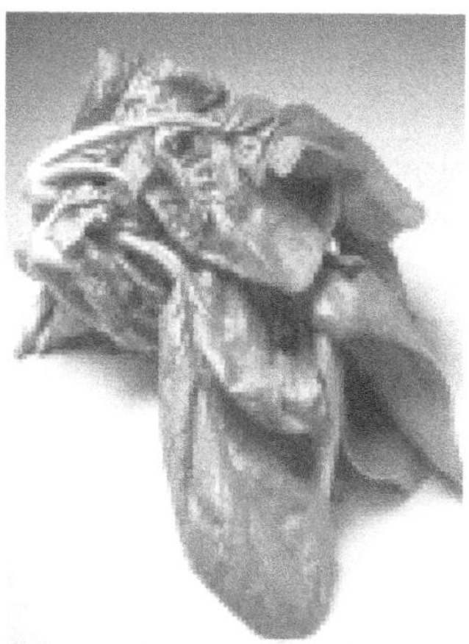

**Ans** Vegetables are natural sources of essential and valuable nutrients. Green leafy vegetables such as spinach, lettuce, cabbage etc. contain a small percentage of solid nutrient. They are rich in alkaline mineral salts, especially soda, lime and iron. They exert a salutatory influence on the composition of the blood by increasing its alkalinity.

Juices obtained from green leafy vegetables such as spinach, cucumber, lettuce, celery and cabbage are no less nutritious than fruit juices. Vegetable juices ignite and promote appetite and for this purpose its intake should proceed before diet.

**Q76. Can one use Coriander leaves in food?**

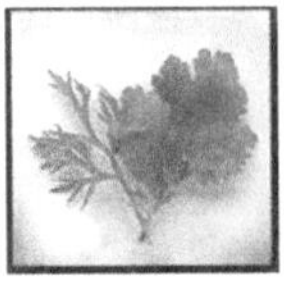

**Ans** Yes, everyone can use Coriander in food. Coriander leaves are pungent leaves, which are used in curries, salads and sauces. In herbalism, small fresh bunches are eaten as a tonic for the stomach and heart. Fresh juice can be used in vitamin deficiency, anemia and constipation, leaves of coriander strengthen the stomach and promote its action. They relieve flatulence, increase secretion and discharge of urine and reduce fever.

**Q77. Can one use Lettuce leaf in Salad?**

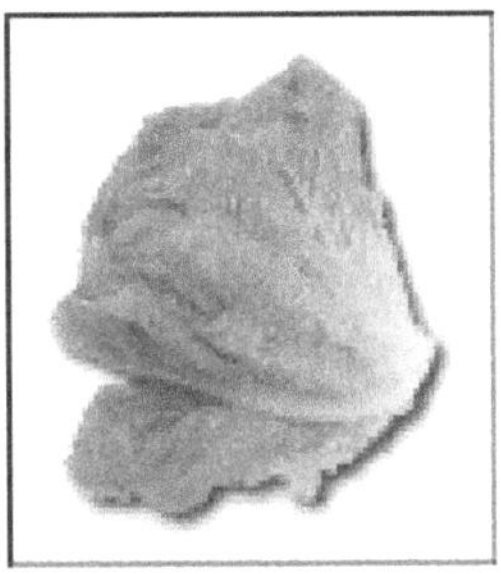

**Ans** Yes, one can use lettuce leaf in salad as they are low in calories, they can be helpful as part of a weight reducing diet provided that they are not coated in fatty salad dressing such as mayonnaise. Lettuce leaves are also a useful source of the antioxidant nutrient beta- carotene, which may help to prevent degenerative disease such as cancer and atherosclerosis. They are a rich source of folate, very low in calories and more than 90% water, they provide nutrients including vitamin C, beta- carotene folate, calcium and iron.

# OTHER VEGETABLES

**Q78. Can I eat Karela/Bitter gourd?**

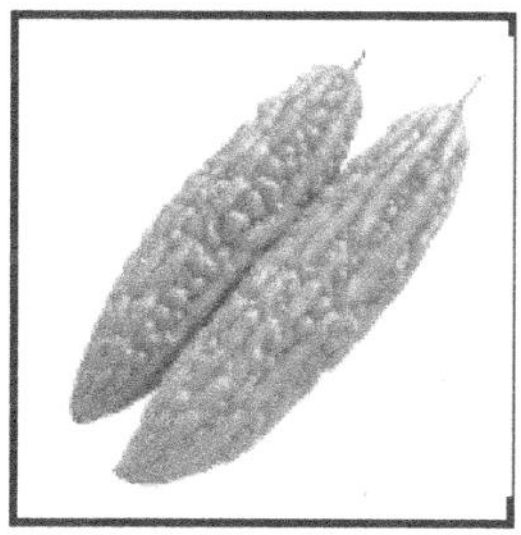

**Ans** Yes, you can eat bitter gourd. Bitter gourd is the only vegetable, which is bitter in taste but it has various beneficial effect. It cures and prevents fever and antidotes of wrong eating's. It is tonic, stomachic, appeasing, laxative and antibilious. It has 'plant insulin factor' which helps in lowering sugar in blood and urine. The diabetic should take 120-140ml juice of fresh bitter gourd on empty stomach, in the morning daily but the same time, keeping a watch over sugar level. A teaspoonful of its powder should be taken with fresh water daily, once or twice, to control diabetes.

It is equally beneficial for various skin and blood disorders like scabies, proriasis, itching, ringworms and other fungal infections as it has been regarded as a great blood purifier. It also anti dotes and detoxifies bad effects of alcohol like damage of liver and digestive disorder.

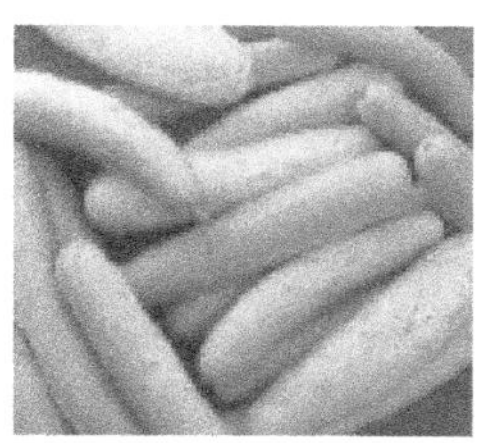

**Q79. Why Lauki juice is considered good for the heart?**

Ans Lauki juice has various beneficial qualities. The juice which is extracted after grating the whole fruit serves as a safeguard against heart conditions, quenches thirst, moistens dry mouth dehydration caused by loose motions, prevents excessive loss of sodium from the body, prevents fatigue. If 5ml of lime juice is added to lauki juice and taken once a day, it will remove the burning sesation in the urine which is caused by high amount of acidity in the urine.

Its cooked vegetable has diuretic, sedative, antibilious and cooling effect on the body. Its vegetable gives a sense of relaxation and satisfaction.

**Q80. Why Tomato is good for heart?**

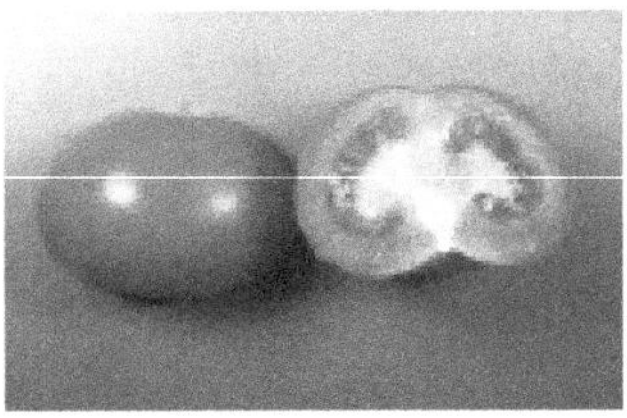

**Ans** Tomato is said to be good for heart because it contains nicotinic acid, which is believed to reduce cholesterol and the vitamin-K is an antihaemorrhagic. Tomato is believed to be natural antiseptic and protects against infections. Tomato juice is a rapid alkalizer and valuable in helping to keep the gums and capillaries firm and well toned. On account of its richness in vitamins and its remineralizing and antitoxic qualities it has a great therapeutic value in arthritis and purification of the blood.

**Q81. Can I take Carrots?**

**Ans** Yes, you can take carrots but you should not be diabetic. It is rich in sulfur, chlorine and sodium and also has traces of iodine. Carrot leaves are highly rich in minerals, protein and vitamins. Due to its rich nutritional values, it is called "A poor man's apple". It is healing, nourishing and soothing, builds up fresh blood and also purifies it. Its raw juice reduces blood cholesterol. Jam of carrot is an effective remedy for the weak heart.

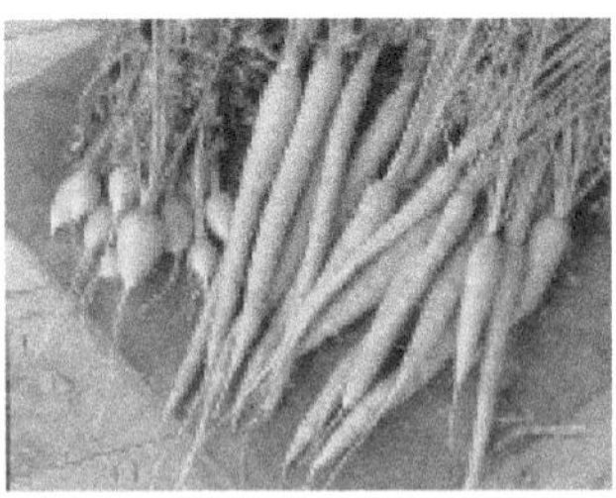

Carrot juice is called a miracle juice. Its juice can effectively control and cure disorders like peptic ulcer, colitis, appendicitis, dyspepsia, intestinal colic, diarrhoea.

**Q82. Can I take Broccoli?**

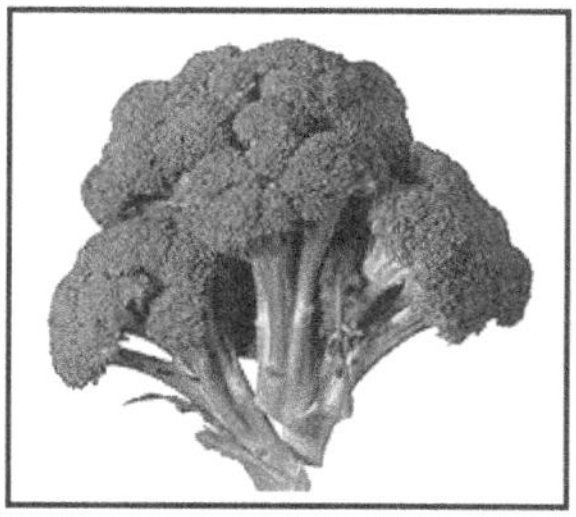

**Ans** Yes, you can eat broccoli. It is a spectacular and unique package of versatile disease fighters, which is abundant in antioxidants- beta-carotene, vitamin-C. It is rich in cholesterol reducing fiber, has antiviral activity, anticancer activity. A super source of chromium helps regulating insulin and blood sugar. It is extremely high in anticancer activity, particularly against lung, colon and breast cancers.

**Q83. Can we take Salads during dinner time?**

**Ans** Yes, you can take salads as much as you want and at any time. But one thing you should keep in mind is that you should not be underweight. If you are underweight you will tend to loose more weight. It provide rich source of fiber and provide bulk to the diet and also helps in elimination of dietary cholesterol and sugar.

**Q84. What if a particular Salad gives me gas?**

**Ans.** Salads produce gas because they are partially digested in the stomach and is not broken down completely and thus produces gas. In such cases avoid such salads, which produce gas (cauliflower, radish etc). If you are eating them make sure you eat methi seeds or saunf.

# FRUITS

## Q85. Can I take Jamun? Is it good for diabetics?

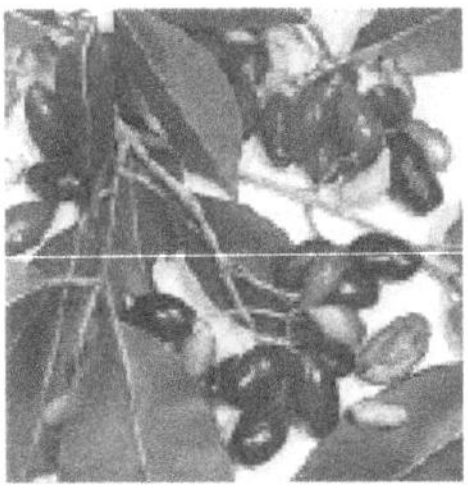

**Ans.** Yes, you can take Jamun. Jamun is also known as black berry. It is known for its hypoglycemic effect. It has specific effect on pancreas and sugar metabolism, which helps in reducing blood sugar levels. It is also claimed and propagated that 3gms powder of jambul seeds, taken thrice daily with water, reduce and allay the unquenched thirst and also reduce quantity of sugar in urine.

## Q86. Can Pineapple be taken?

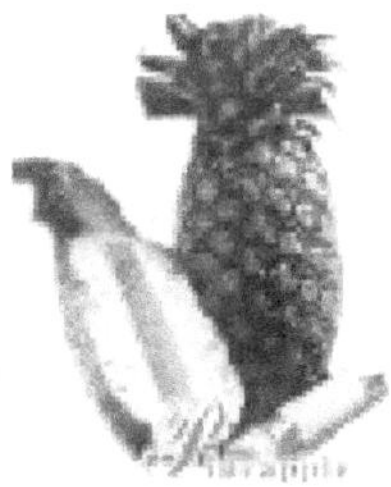

**Ans** Yes pineapple can be taken if you are not diabetic. It is a delicious and healthy fruit. It has a high fiber content, which helps in reducing cholesterol levels. It also has many other beneficial qualities like raising the alkaline reserve of the blood in case of edema by getting rid of excess of water in the system. It also helps in cough and bronchitis.

## Q87. Can Papaya be taken by heart patients?

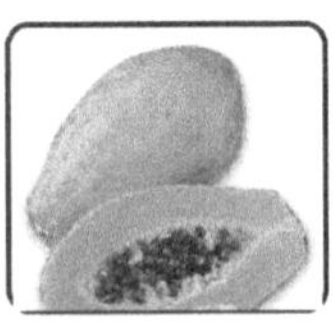

**Ans** Yes heart patients can take papaya. Even diabetic patients can eat papaya it but should not be sweet to the tongue. Papaya is a rich source of vitamins A,C and iron. It is easily digestible and provides energy to the body and also helps in removing constipation. It also has soluble fiber, which helps in cholesterol reduction.

**Q88. Can heart patients eat Lichie?**

**Ans.** Heart patients can eat lichie but it cannot be eaten by diabetics. It is a good summer fruit with fresh and juicy pulp.

**Q89. Why doctors suggest eating Guava?**

**Ans.** Guava is a rich source of vitamin C. Doctors suggest it because it is a good cholesterol lowering agent and have laxative properties. It has soluble fiber, which also helps in reduction of blood sugar levels.

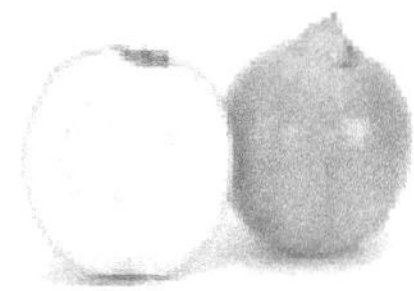

**Q90. What all fruits should be avoided by heart patients those who are obese and diabetic?**

**Ans** Banana, mango, grapes, cheeku are the fruits which should be avoided by the heart patients those whose are diabetic.

**Q91. Which is good fresh fruits or fruit juice?**

**Ans** Fresh fruits are a better option than fruit juice. The advantage lies in high amount of fiber, which is present in whole fruits and is absent in fruit juice. Fruits have both soluble and insoluble fiber. The insoluble fiber helps to prevent constipation and is associated with a reduced risk of colon cancer, while the soluble fiber can help to lower blood cholesterol level and the fruit juice lacks in only this property of fruits i.e., all the fiber is destroyed or thrown as waste product.

**Q92. Is peeling of the fruits a good practice?**

**Ans.** Peeling of the fruits before eating is not a good practice as peeling of covers means peeling out all the fiber of the fruits. But some fruits cannot be eaten without peeling like banana, papaya.

**Q93. Why Amla is considered good for heart patients?**

**Ans.** It is an indigenous fruit of India and is the richest sources of natural vitamin C, which is easily assimilated by the human body. In whichever form it is eaten / consumed its contents of vitamin C never get depleted. It is also the best of all acid fruits and is used freely and often in disease and health. It is of unquestioned use and value for various defects in the body and heart.

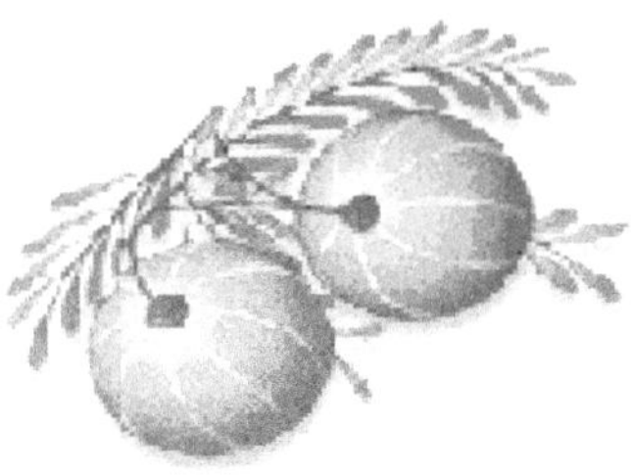

It is of immense value, if used in diabetes, heart disease, respiratory disorders, eye disorders, scurvy, loose motions and dysentery for retarding and preventive aging or for health of hair. There is hardly any organ, rather none of the human body, which does not derive benefit from the use of amla, either alone or in combination with other ingredients. In the treatment of diarrhoea and dysentery, prepare a paste of leaves of berry and mix buttermilk or honey to 15 ml of paste. Dried fruit powder is also useful for the said two disorders. But to control acute dysentery, prepare a drink made from mixing amla juice/ powder with sugar candy and lemon juice.

Amla strengthens, rejuvenates, builds up damaged tissue of the body removes wrinkles and blemishes. For diabetic patients, 15 ml of its fresh juice should be added to a cup of fresh juice of bitter gourd to be taken daily in the morning and evening for two months will stimulate Islets of Langerhans, thus reducing sugar in the blood. As an alternative mix up equal quantity of powders of jambul, amla and bitter gourd and take a tablespoon each thrice daily to yield desired results. The said recipes are capable of preventing any eye problem, which appears as a consequence of diabetes.

# NUTS AND OILSEEDS

## Q94. Can I take Dates?

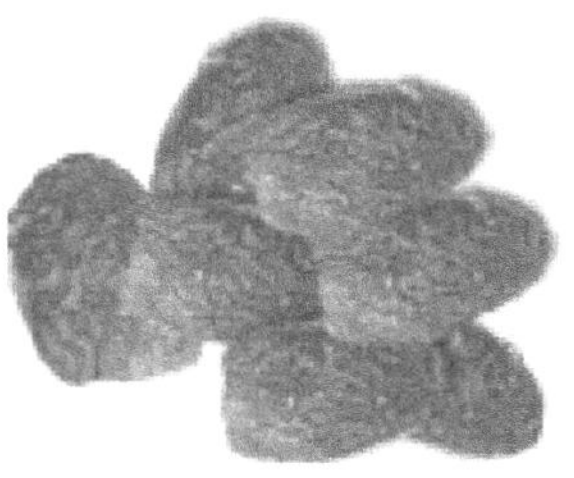

**Ans.** Yes, you can take dates. The value of dates from the health point of view is superb. It is wholesome, easily digested and assimilated and energizing. Dates contain a very high percentage of sugar in natural form, which is immediately absorbed. They are rich in protein, iron, vitamins and other essential food constituents, which are a wholesome substitute for a cane sugar. Dates are frequently eaten raw and are a good substitute for candy and sweets for children. The powdered date seeds are used in cooking, as they are rich in starch and fats. If you are not diabetic you can take dates. 100gm of dates will provide you with 317 cal. Since they are providing this much of calories so if you are over weight or obese you should count your calories well.

## Q95. Can I take Figs(Angeer)?

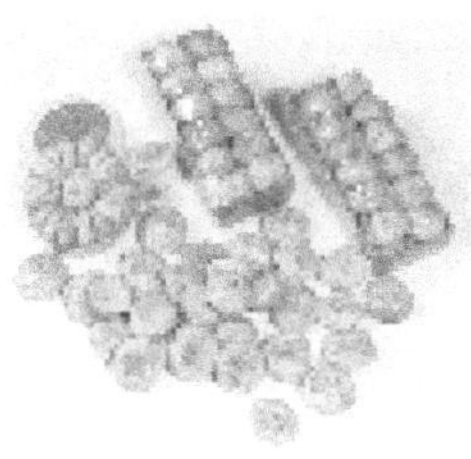

**Ans** Yes, you can take dried fig. The dried fig is rich in sugar and contains calcium and protein. It is considered most effective in counteracting constipation especially when soaked overnight in water. The dried black fig is popular as a health food and is a highly nutritious. If not diabetic 100gms of fresh figs will give you 317 cal. Figs are great health promoters and easily digestible. Sugar content of dry figs is high.

**Q96. Can I take Almonds(Badam)?**

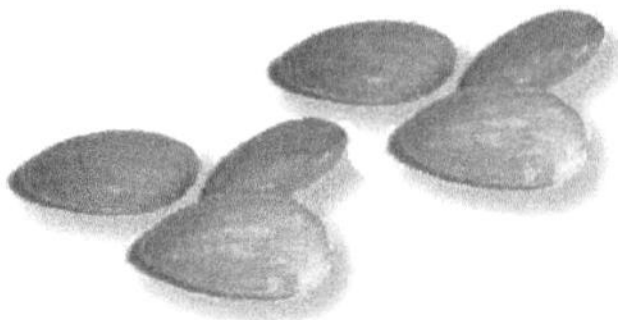

**Ans.** Almonds are the seeds of a tree closely related to the peach in fact the fruits look rather like a small green peaches.

There are two basic varieties of almonds – Sweet Almonds and Bitter almonds.

Sweet Almonds have an inimitable, delicate flavour. It is this type, which is usually used in cooking.

Bitter Almonds are similar to that of the kernels of plums, peaches, cherries and other related fruits. They are bitter in taste and are toxic to body if children below 10 yrs eat them it is threat to life.

Almonds are extremely nourishing and have long been valued as a good muscle – and body building substance. They are high in fat, carbohydrate and protein and their calcium content is particularly valuable for building children's teeth and bones. Intake of 100 gm of almonds will give 58.9 gm of fat, which means 12 tsp full of oil. Also they contain little starch and so invaluable in the diet of person suffering from diabetes.

**Q97. Can I take Cashew nut(Kaju)?**

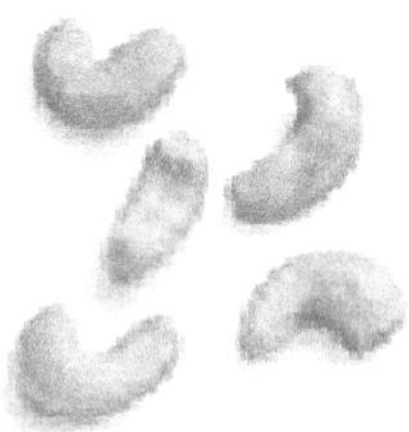

**Ans.** No, you cannot have cashew nut. Cashew nut is white, sweet and kidney shaped and extremely versatile as far as its culinary uses are concerned, capable of being salted, roasted, creamed, made into liquor or used cashew nut are good body builders and easily digested when raw and so help in cases of emaciation and in building good teeth. Boiling them in oil or salting them makes them harder to digest so they are best eaten in their natural state. They can go best with acid fruit and non-starchy vegetables rather than sweet fruit and heavy starch.

Like all nuts cashews contain a great deal of unsaturated fatty acid, mostly in the form of oleic acid. On consumption of 100gms of cashew nuts you will give 47 gm of fat. Almost 9 teaspoon full of oil you are going to put in your body.

## Q98. Can I take Raisins and Munnaka?

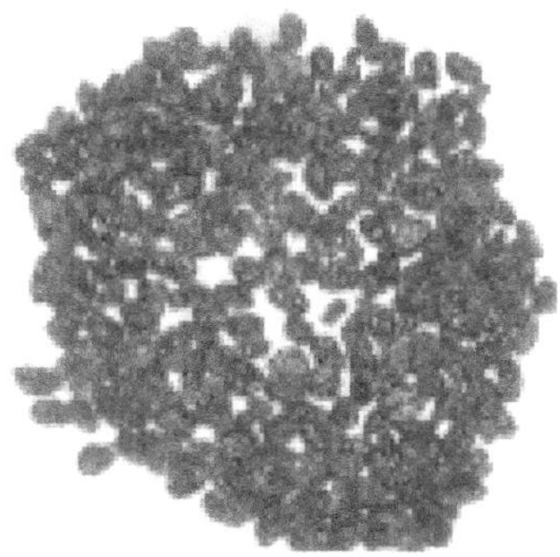

**Ans.** Yes, you can take raisins but moderately. Raisins are among those fruits and vegetables, which enjoy the greatest predominance of alkalinity. The outstanding value or raisins in relieving acidosis is because of their striking quality.

In raisins three fourths of the dry weight of the fruits is in the form of pure fruit sugar, emphasizing their importance, as a quick energy food. 100 gm of each will give you 308 cal.

Munnaka (prunes) have been highly recommended for combating constipation but should be used sparingly and must be avoided by those who suffer from gout, uric acid and a tendency to acidosis as they contain benzoic acid, which tends to render tissue fluids and the urine, acid. It is said that there is a certain medicinal property in the prune, which acts directly upon the nervous system. It seems to posses a soothing property, which calms the mind and removes nervous irritability. Heart patient can take munnaka but in small quantities as they are high calorie foods 316 cal respectively. Therefore, three fourth of dry weight is in the form of pure sugar so they should be avoided by diabetics.

### Q99. Can I take Pista?

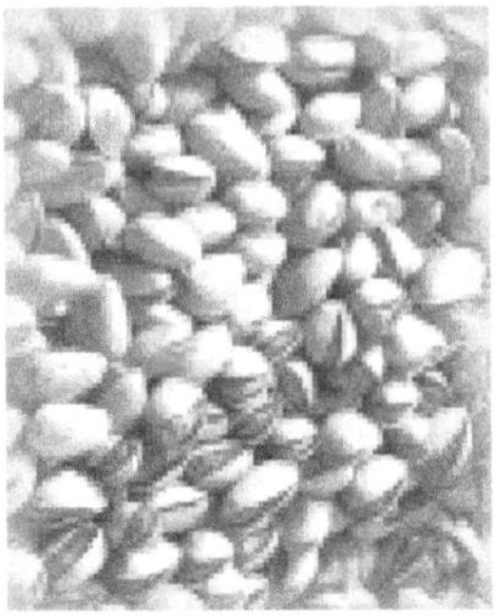

**Ans.** No, you cannot take pista as it is rich in Triglycerides. The kernel of the pistachio nut is covered with thin brown red skin but the flesh of kernel is bright green. In general, the greener the colour of pista better the quality.

Pistachio nuts are a good source of protein and contain several vitamins including A and B1. They are fairly rich in potassium and phosphorus and have small amounts of iron and calcium. But because they are rich in Triglycerides they have to be avoided, as they are the primary cause for blockages.

### Q100. Can I take Walnut (Akhrot)?

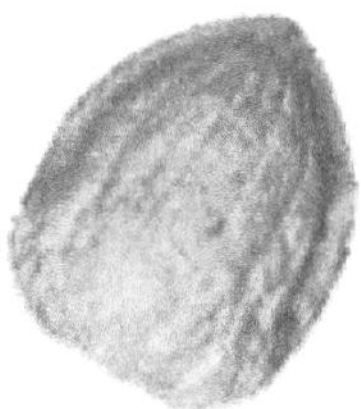

**Ans.** Walnut resembles the human brain and is usually eaten. The shells are thin with a faint sheen and crack neatly in half, revealing the twisted, curly shaped nut. Walnuts are barely ripe have a very delicate flavor.

Walnuts are very rich in protein and also contain a small amount of vitamin B. they should be eaten in small quantities and go well with fruits.

They have a curative value in cases of eczema. Oil obtained from the kernel has been found of great help in skin diseases. The green unripe walnut is useful for expelling worms. They are said to be good for constipation as they have a definite laxative effect. But above all this they are very high calorie foods. Though walnuts are rich in protein. They are effective in some skin diseases. But above all this they are very high calorie food and more over 100 gms of walnut gives 64.5 gms of fat. This will definitely increase Triglyceride and so should be restricted.

## Q101. Can I take Coconut and Coconut Milk?

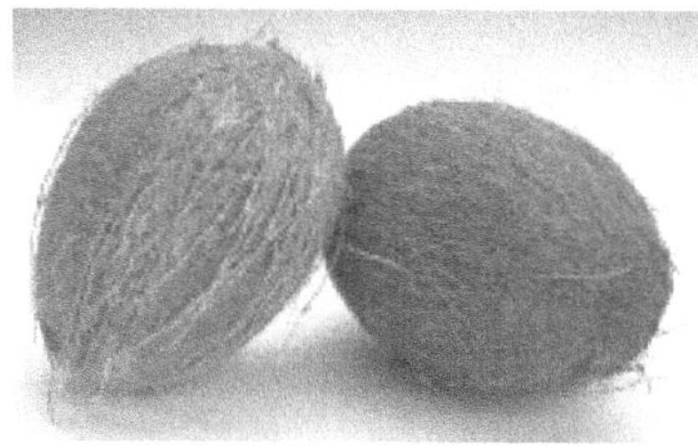

**Ans** The coconut is considered to be very close to a perfect food, containing all the elements necessary for the proper nutrition of the human body. This tropical "wonder food" is rich in vitamin A, B1. It is a valuable source of potassium, sodium, calcium, magnesium, iron, phosphorus and sulphur. The carbohydrates and protein content of coconut are moderate. It is one of the finest vegetable oil containing food. The fat content is high and of course useful as it furnishes the body with a natural and abundant supply of the finest lubricant. Coconut water is diuretic and can be used against any kind of fever. It is a cleaner of the kidneys and gall bladder. Coconut is a very popular food in Indian cooking specially in South India it is used in almost every dish. But the fact is that nobody is aware of high fat content in coconut 100 gm of fresh coconut will give you 41.6 gm of fat and 100gms of dry coconut (Copra) will give you 62.3 gms of fat and composition of 100gms of coconut oil is 1% poly unsaturated fatty acid, 8% of mono unsaturated fatty acid and 91% of saturated fatty acid. So a heart patient cannot have coconut or coconut milk at all.

## Q102. Can I take Poppy Seeds?

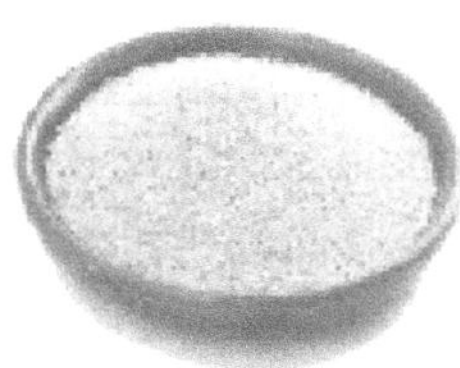

**Ans** Yes, poppy seeds can be used but in moderate quantities. Poppy seeds are sweet in flavour and used in cookery. It is an important source of oils. The part of the poppy most used for medicinal purposes is the petals of the corn poppy and the capsules of the opium poppy. The seeds have been used to treat intestinal disorders and to keep the bowl movement regular.

They are tiny dark cream colour seeds of poppy plant, which

are used for topping of bread, cake, rolls or filling of buns. Oil extract is used for salads. Poppy seeds are used as thickening agent in the preparation of gravies.

Poppy seeds are usually used in sweet dish preparation. They also make a part in many sweet drinks like Thandai.

### Q103. Can I take Mustard Seeds(Rai)?

**Ans** Yes, you can eat mustard seeds but it should be taken moderately. They are the small reddish black seeds of annual herbs. The leaves of this plant are consumed as vegetable. Mustard seeds have a pungent flavour. It is used in the vegetable preparation and raita. It is used mainly for the seasoning. Mustard is used without the skin for pickling. Mustard oil is used in cookery.

The pungent taste and tear, producing properties of mustard seeds are due to nitrogen and sulphur containing compounds called isothiocynates. Mustard seeds are used in treating rheumatism, arthritis, and acidity. Kidney and bladder ailments and bronchial inflammation and are recommended particularly for pregnant women and nursing mothers, to rid the system of accumulated poisons. Mustard greens are rich in vitamin A, B and C and contain bulk fiber, which produces a mildly laxative effect. It should be taken sparingly internally because it can cause inflammation.

### Q104. Can I take Fenugreek Seeds(Methi)?

**Ans** Yes, you can take Fenugreek seeds. It is hard lentil seed. Its colour is dark fawn and has astringent aroma. Fenugreek seeds contain 5% bitter fixed oil. The oil has strong celery like odor. It is moderate. It is one of the finest vegetable oil containing food. The fat content is high i.e., 40% that is why it is to be avoided by heart patient as it increases the blood Triglyceride level.

### Q105. Can I eat Groundnut?

**Ans** Being a heart patient you should not consume groundnut in any form. Whether it is roasted, soaked in water or boiled. Though groundnut resemble other pulses in general nutritive value but they are very rich in fat on consuming 100 gms of fat one will get almost 40gm of oil. This is nothing but Triglyceride.

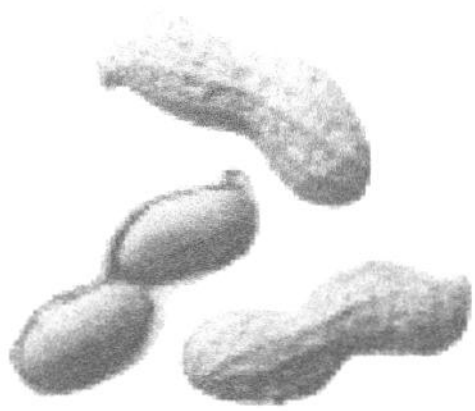

**Q106. Does Almond contain cholesterol?**

**Ans.** No, almond does not contain cholesterol but it contains 58.9% fat i.e. Triglycerides which increases the blood level of Triglyceride and thus causing the hardening of the arteries. Being the "King of Nuts" all its nutritional value becomes zero because of its fat content.

**Q107. Can dry Coconut be taken?**

**Ans.** No, dry coconut cannot be taken. This tropical wonder food is rich in vitamins A, B and C. It is a valuable source of potassium, sodium, calcium, magnesium, iron, phosphorus and sulphur. The carbohydrates and protein contents of coconut are moderate. It is one of the finest vegetable oil containing food. The fat content is high i.e., 40% that is why it is to be avoided by heart patient as it increases the blood Triglyceride level.

## SPICES

**Q108. Can I put Garam Masala in my vegetable?**

**Ans** Is there any oil in garam masala? No, so no restriction on the use of garam masala in vegetables. It is only restricted for those who have some gastric problem or those who are or had suffered from ulcers any time in their life.

**Q109. Can I consume Red Chillies and Chilli powder?**

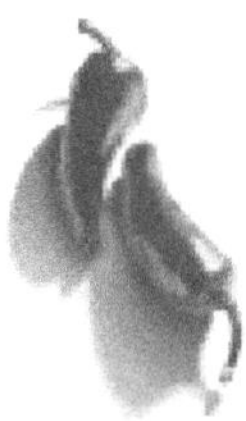

**Ans** Yes, you can have chillies but they should be taken in very less quantity as they may cause burning sensation. Chillies have always been used as a flavouring agent in dishes. They make a bland food spicy and hot. There is no harm in consuming red chillies and chilli powder by heart patients.

**Q110. Can I use Sambar Masala?**

**Ans** A heart patient can use Sambar masala provided the masala is prepared at home. During the preparation of Sambar masala in the market some masalas are fried in oil before they are grinded. This frying should be avoided at home.

**Q111. Can I take Tamarind?**

**Ans** Yes you can take tamarind. Tamarind is widely used in Indian cooking as souring agent. It makes a very important place in dishes like chutneys, chaats, pickles, sambar etc. Tamarind is rich in vitamin-C which is an antioxidant and so good for heart.

**Q112. Can I use Ginger?**

**Ans** Yes, you can use Ginger. It is being used in India from

vedic period as mahaushadi, meaning the great medicine. It has been used for centuries to treat a variety of diseases like nausea, vomiting, headache, chest congestion, cholera, colds, diarrhoea, stomachache and nervous diseases. It is a powerful anti-oxidant. It also ranks very high in anti-cancer activities.

**Q113. Can I use Asafoetida (Hing)?**

**Ans** Yes, you can use asafoetida in your food. It has properties to expel wind from the stomach and counteract many spasmodic disorders. It is also a nervine stimulant, digestive agent and a sedative. It has antibiotic properties and inhibits growth of microbes.

**Q114. Can I use Clove?**

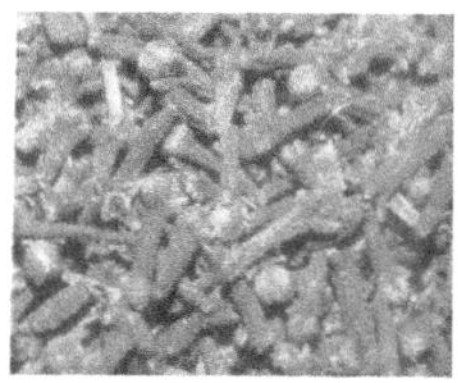

**Ans** Yes, you can use clove. It has many medicinal properties. These properties emanate from volatile oil contained in it. It is stimulant, carminative, antiseptic, antispasmodic and expectorant. It also helps to stimulate sluggish circulation and metabolism.

**Q115. Can I use Pepper?**

**Ans** Yes, you can use black pepper. It is a stimulant, pungent, aromatic, digestive and nervine tonic. The pungency of pepper is due to the resin chavicine. Black pepper is useful in relieving flatulence and it is known as "king of spices".

**Q116. Can we put Tej Patta in vegetables?**

**Ans** Yes, you can use Tej Patta comes under spices and saaol puts restriction on intake of oil and not on spices so a heart patient can have Tej Patta in vegetables.

# ROOTS AND TUBERS

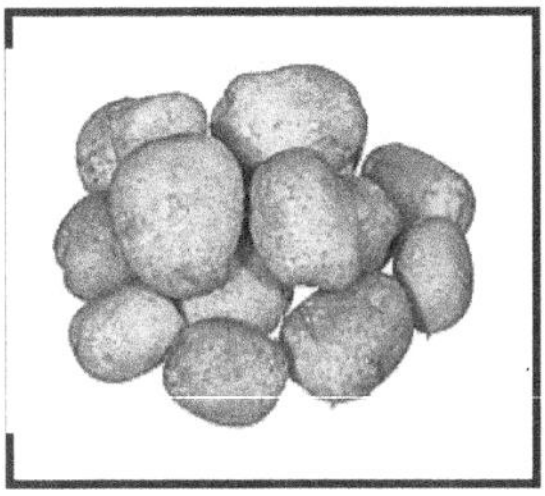

**Q117. Can I eat Potato?**

**Ans** Yes, you can eat potato but it should be eaten moderately. Potato is one of the staple foods. Next to cereals potatoes are considered to be the most important food. They are valuable chiefly because they contain a very digestive starch and secondly because they offer a rich variety of mineral salts The great value of the potato as a good lies in the fact, that at a very low cost, it furnishes an abundance of carbohydrates, high calories, with a small amount of mineral elements. It is rich in potassium, silicon, sodium and magnesium. Raw potatoes are an excellent source of vitamin C and a fair amount of vitamin B.

**Q118. What is the benefit of eating Onion?**

**Ans** Onions are mild acid neutralizers. They are rich in vitamin C, good in B and fair in A. Raw onions are excellent natural digestive stimulants. They contain a hormone, which promotes the intestinal secretions of endocrine glands. They are also considered a good aphrodisiac. They have a fair source of organic calcium, potassium, iron, phosphorus, magnesium, sulfur, also a little sodium and chlorine. They are specially rich in organic silicon and have a strong antiseptic effect. It is said that onion is instrumental in normalizing percentages of blood cholesterol by oxidizing the excess cholesterol and also has a specific action in atherosclerosis. It is therefore, useful as a prophylaxis in cardio vascular disorders. One teaspoon of raw onion juice on rising is supposed to be excellent for heart disease and blood cholesterol.

The onion is carminative, diuretic, stimulant, and anti inflammatory anti spasmodic stimulant to the circulatory system and anticoagulant. It is an antiseptic of high potency. It is good for nerves, anemia and insomnia. Raw onions are powerful antiseptic they also attract disease germs and poison to themselves.

**Q119 Is there any harm in taking Jimikand/Yam?**

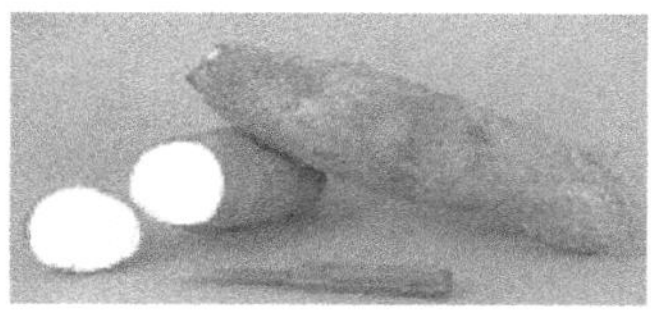

**Ans** No, there is no harm in taking yam. But it should be consumed moderately specially by diabetics. Yam is a rich source of starch and provide high calorie. 100gm of boiled yam provides 133 calories. Yam is a good source of potassium needed for muscle and nerve function and the yellow-fleshed varieties can be useful source of calories. It is to be avoided by overweight but underweight can consume freely to increase their weight.

**Q120 Can I eat Beetroot?**

**Ans** Yes, you can eat beetroot but moderately. It is a rich source of natural sugar. Best way, to use it is to use its fresh juice, which has plenty of potassium, sodium, phosphorus chlorine, sulfur, iron, iodine, copper and Vitamins like B-1, B-2, B-6, C and Niacin, and is easily digestible. Though it is high in Carbohydrates, it is low in calorific content. Besides it has also amino acids in quantity and quality, beetroot should not be consumed during summer, as it may push up blood pressure. Beetroot has cellulose content which acts as a bulking agent. It eases smooth passage of stool and prevents constipation.

# SUGAR

## Q121. Can I take Sugar?

**Ans** Yes, you can take sugar but in a very limited quantity. especially diabetics should avoid sugar as sugar can instantly raise their blood sugar level. One can always make use of jaggery instead of sugar. Over weight people should also avoid as it provides high calories.

## Q122. Can I take Jaggery?

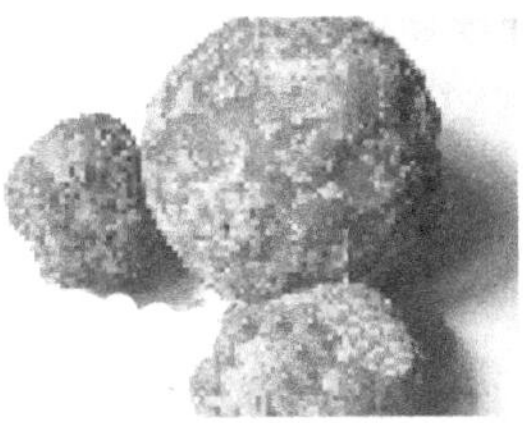

**Ans** Yes, you can take jaggery. Jaggery is obtained mainly from cane syrup. It can also be obtained from palm and date. It is always recommended to take jaggery in place of sugar. Jaggery is preferred to sugar because it is rich in iron requires less refining as compared to sugar and it is less expensive.

## Q123. Can I take Honey?

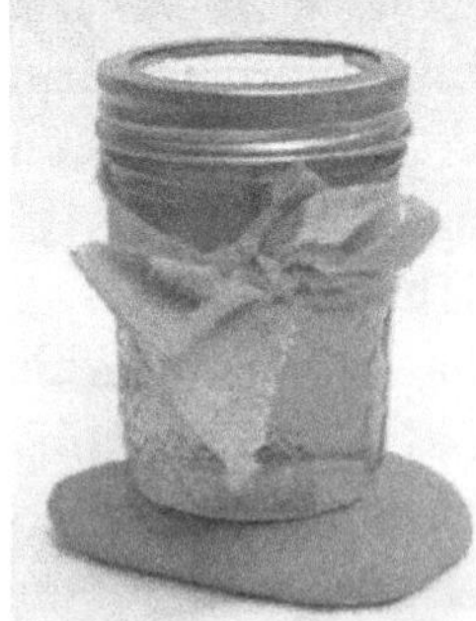

**Ans** Yes, you can take honey but diabetics should avoid it to some extent. Honey is a tonic for the body as it has immense food values consisting of 28 minerals, 11 enzymes, 22 amino acids, 14 fatty acids. It has unique food values and medicinal properties. It is yellowish- brown in Colour, semi – translucent, having viscid, and is too sweet. Basic sugars remains constant in honey at 76% (approx) since it contain sucrose – 2%, levulose – 40% and dextrose – 34%, dextrine and gums range from 1.5 to 2%. Honey is digested within twenty minutes of its intake. It is far more superior to other forms of sugar.

Honey and lemon juice should be mixed in lukewarm water to reduce weight and should be taken in the morning on empty stomach. The thin and weak persons should take two teaspoon of honey mixed in warm milk in the morning or at bedtime to gain weight and strength.

For cough and colds equal quantity of fresh juice of basil & ginger be mixed with honey and licked. Whenever you feel tired and exhausted, take 10 – 15ml of honey in water. Honey reduce uric acid, hence it is useful in gouty and rheumatic cases. It is equally useful for arthritis also. Honey helps to subside pains and swelling due to burns. Honey is used in any form, is an infallible food item.

### Q124. What is Equal? Is it safe to take?

**Ans** Equal or sugar free are commercially available artificial sweetners. They are chemicals, which can stimulate our sweet sensitive taste buds. They can be used to make sweets for diabetic heart patients. They have another advantage that they do not have calories. It can be taken by heart patients for loosing weight (by replacing sugar in diet). So far no side effects have been reported about aspartame. A maximum of 6-10 tablets/day can be taken.

### Q125. Can Saccharine/Sweetex be taken instead of Equal?

**Ans** Yes, you can take Saccharine/Sweetex instead of Equal. Actually there is no difference between them the difference lies only in their chemical formula. Saccharine should be avoided as it is proved to be carcinogenic instead you can take aspartame. Artificial sweetners are chief coaltar products, substituted for sugar. Being extremely sweet they are much used by certain manufacturers also in aerated waters and by persons suffering from diabetes.

# SAUCE AND CHUTNEYS

## Q126. Can I eat Tomato Sauce?

**Ans** Tomato sauce is a mixture tomato, onion, garlic and sugar, salt, garam masala and preservatives like sodium benzoate and acetic acid.

Heart patients can easily take tomato sauce, as it doesn't have any oil. But if a patient is diabetic also then it should be made in home i.e. home made preparation by having sugar free instead of sugar.

Best way is to cook tomato sauce in home or take fresh tomato chutney as we can make it, according to our limitations and medical condition.

## Q127. Can heart patient take Chutneys?

Ans Heart patient can take all the chutneys except coconut as it contain 40% of oil so it is to be avoided by heart patients. Other chutneys which heart patients can consume freely are –

Dhania pudina chutney – one bunch dhania, half bunch mint, a little roasted bengalgram and urad dal, 2 chillies, salt to taste, 2 table spoon curd (of skimmed milk) Grind all the ingredients.

Curry leaves chutney– One bunch curry leaves, a little roasted urad dal and 2 red chillies, one or half tomato salt to taste. Grind all the ingredients coarse with less water. This chutney can be mixed with rice.

Carrot chutney– boiled or cooked carrots 1 cup, 2 chillies, salt to taste. Wash and grind all ingredients fine. Serve with any snack.

### Q128. Can I take Pickle?

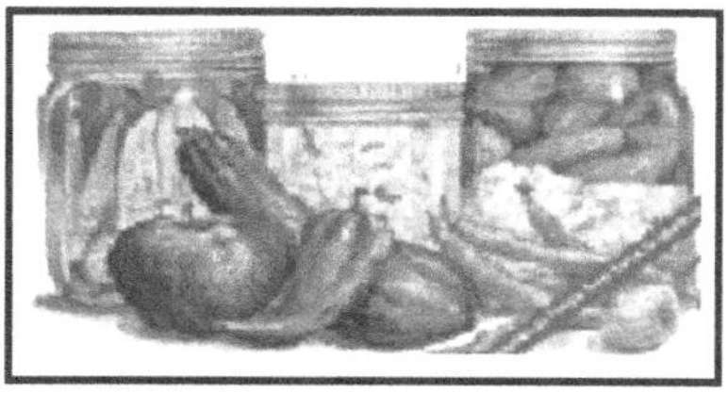

**Ans** Yes, you can eat pickles but they should not contain any oil. Pickling is a traditional way of preserving fresh fruit and vegetables by discouraging the growth of microbes that would otherwise cause them to decompose. People on low salt diet should try to avoid pickle because of their high sodium content. Pickles and chutneys can also trigger allergies.

Heart patient can take any pickle made without a single drop of oil like- Mirchi pickle, Amla ka achar, Aam ka achaar, Mix vegetable pickle, lemon pickle. These pickles are made by the use of vinegar, sodium benzoate as a preservative. The important thing to be kept in mind is that these pickles should not be stored for a very long time as there shelf life is very less, Now in market all the varieties of pickle without oil is available.

### Q129. Can I take Jam?

**Ans** Yes, you can take jam but diabetic and overweight heart patients should avoid jams. Jams offer little more than concentrated energy in the form of sugar. One tablespoon contains around 40 calories. Jam contributes minute amounts of dietary fiber in the form of pectin and only little amount of vitamins. The heat treatment involved in the boiling of preserves greatly reduces their vitamins content.

### Q130. Can I take Jellies?

**Ans** Yes, you can eat jellies but remember you should not be diabetic. Jellies are made up of clear fruit juice. Gelatin is added to set the jellies. Sugar is added, as a preservative so diabetic patients should avoid jellies.

# TEA AND COFFEE

### Q131. Can I take Coffee?

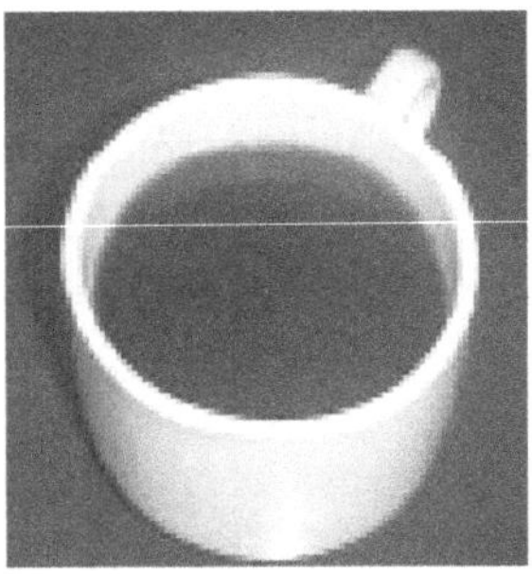

**Ans** Yes, you can take coffee but not more than 2 cups per day. Coffee is a stimulating beverage. Its stimulating properties being due to the presence of an active alkaloid principal known as caffeine, have a marked effect upon the action of the heart and preventing sleep.

Coffee is prepared from the seeds of the coffee tree. The aroma and flavour of coffee is due to a volatile oil, which is liberated on roasting the hard, almost tasteless bean to a high temperature. The best way to make coffee is by the filter or percolator. Being a stimulating beverage it has been suggested not to drink coffee daily as it is a habit-forming drug.

### Q132. Can I take Tea?

**Ans** Yes, you can take tea but not more than two cups a day.

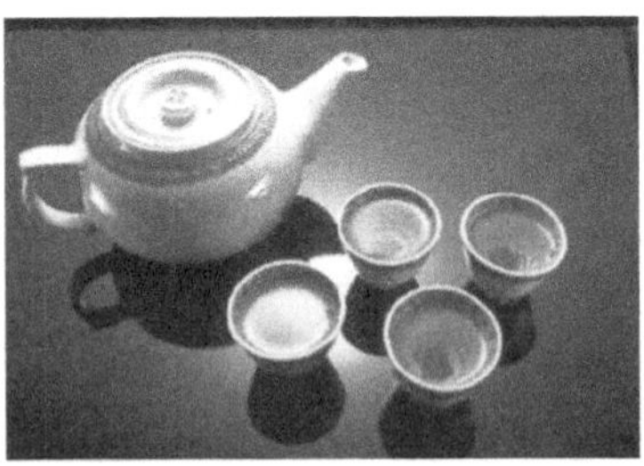

Recent research has found that black tea consumption may lower bad cholesterol levels and could one day be used to help reduce the chance of heart disease. Green tea is another tea, which is beneficial. It is also called herbal tea. Actually SAAOL does not recommend tea for more than 2 cups a day because it has got antinutrients. These antinutrients do not allow nutrients to get absorbed in the body. So tea should be taken in limited quantity. SAAOL only recommends SAAOL tea, which has many herbs in it including Arjuna Barkhich helps in reduction of blood cholesterol.

## DRINKS

### Q133. Can I drink Soft drinks?

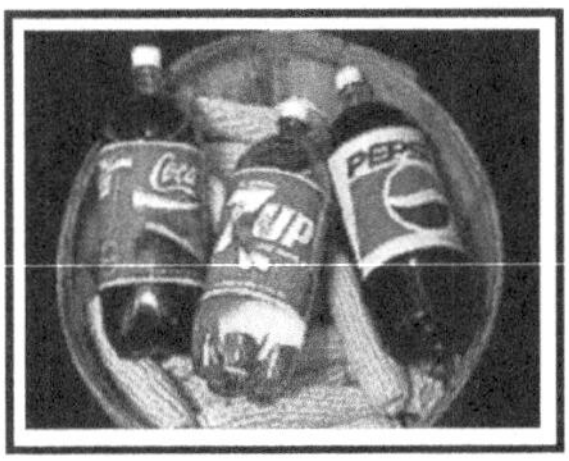


**Ans** Yes, you can drink soft drinks but it should be taken moderately. Diabetic heart patients should avoid these drinks. Most sweetened soft drinks provide empty calories, but no other useful nutrients.

### Q134. What are low calorie drinks?

**Ans** Low calorie drinks are made with artificial sweetners. Low calorie drinks are suitable for almost everyone, including diabetics. They do not contribute to tooth decay by promoting the formation of plague, or to weight problems. Sparkling waters with added herbs, minerals and ginseng claim to act as a natural pick up, but tend to be more expensive than other soft drinks. They are usually sweetened with fruit juice.

### Q135. What drinks a heart patient can take?

**Ans** Drinks, which heart patient, can take are-

- Lemon water
- Lemon soda
- Nutrient dense juices
- Vegetable soup
- Cold drinks

- Instant Soup mixes.
- Frooti

But in these, the drinks, which contain a lot of sugar is to be avoided by diabetics.

**Q136. Can I take Diet Coke?**

**Ans** Yes, you can take diet coke as it contains very less calories i.e.0.9 calories per 200 gram and no sugar.

# SOUPS & JUICES

**Q137. Can heart patients take Non-Vegetarian soups?**

**Ans** No, heart patients cannot take non- vegetarian soup because it contains lot of cholesterol and it will raise the blood cholesterol level.

**Q138. How to increase calorie of Soups?**

**Ans** Calories of soup can be increased by the following ways i.e. by adding

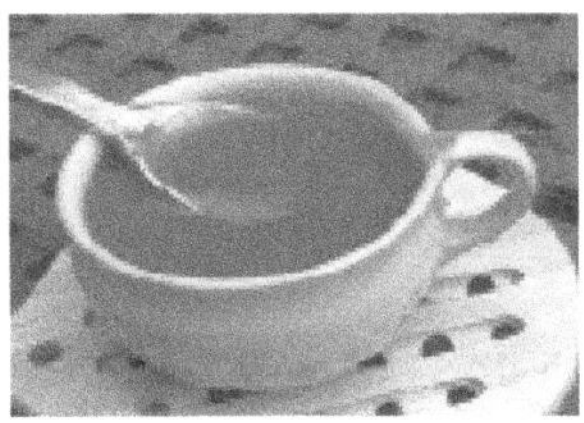

- Corn flour
- Breadcrumbs
- Soya sauce & Vinegar
- Bread pieces

# ALCOHOL AND WINE

**Q139. How is Alcohol bad for the heart?**

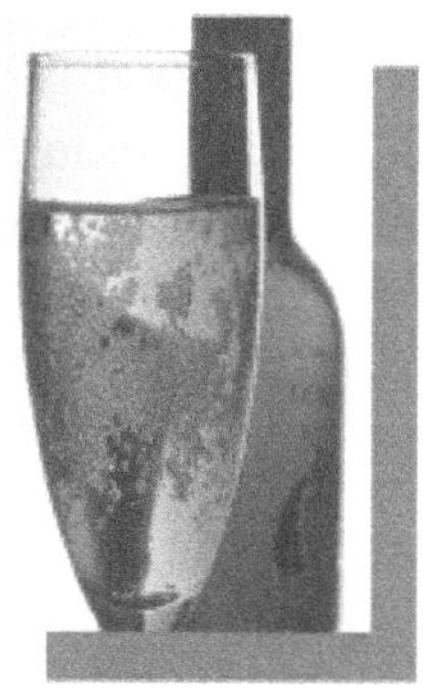

**Ans** While small amounts of alcohol do not harm and may even be beneficial both for cordial social interaction and relaxation, heavy alcohol consumption of more than two ounces of whisky in a day or its equivalent of two glasses of beer or two glasses of wine is harmful not only for the liver and stomach but also for the heart as it results in higher blood pressure and harmful blood fats which are the risk factors for heart attack. Heavy drinking is also responsible for social problems such as traffic accidents, death, divorces, and absence from work.

"There is no minimum threshold below which alcohol can be consumed without any risk. Alcoholism can be blamed for some of the world's most serious problems. The less you drink the better."

**Q140. Can I take Red Wine?**

**Ans** No, a heart patient cannot take red wine. Though all alcohol including red wine increases HDL cholesterol level in blood but they also increase triglyceride level, which are responsible for blockages. So they should be avoided including red wine.

## SALT AND HYPERTENSION

**Q141. Is there any restriction on Salt for heart patients?**

**Ans** There is no restriction on salt for the heart patients. If high blood pressure is associated with heart disease then salt intake should be restricted. A part from this patients with low pumping power should reduce or should restrict salt to below 5gm/day.

# OBESITY AND FOOD

**Q142. What kind of food should be taken for loosing weight?**

1. Follow total vegetarianism.
2. Take skimmed/double toned milk (200-250ml/day)
3. No oil to be used for cooking.
4. Zero oil cooking methods. Use non-stick, pressure-cooking Heating, Baking, Boiling, Roasting
5. Salads before every meal.
6. Prefer brown bread instead of white bread.
7. Avoid raw sugar.
8. Alteration of pulses.
9. Mix wheat bran, soyaflour or besan with wheat flour.
10. Stuff chapaties with green leafy vegetables & wheat bran.
11. Don't use butter on bread instead use dhania, pudina chutney, sauce, jelly, jam.
12. Avoid alcohol.
13. Take soups, lemon water, and fruit juices.
14. Increase intake of whole grains and legumes.
15. Prefer fruits with their skins.
16. Use sprouts.

17. Add boiled vegetables in rice, noodles, and soups.
18. Take more row calorie fruits and avoid the high calorie ones like mango, banana, cheeku, and grapes.
19. Dine at least two hours before you go to bed.
20. Eat to live and don't live to eat.

**Q143. Does obesity or overweight play any role in heart disease?**

**Ans** It has been observed that people who are overweight, that is, those with BMI (Body Mass Index = weight in Kgs divided by Height in square) above 27, have high levels of blood cholesterol and Triglycerides, Low HDL (High Density Lipoprotein) which is the good heart friendly cholesterol and higher blood pressures – all these being the risk factors for Heart Attacks.

# UNDER WEIGHT

**Q144. What kind of food should be taken for gaining weight?**

**Ans** For heart patients we do not recommend any kind of oil – which otherwise contains lot of calories but to gain weight a heart patient must consume more calories/day. Thus we recommend them to consume any thing from 1800-2500 calories/day, but without any oil and cholesterol, the following food is to be consumed in plenty by those who want to gain weight.

- Lots of cereals & pulses.
- Egg white.
- Sweets made without oil.
- Soft drinks.
- Banana.

They should avoid low calorie food like:-

- Salad
- Low calorie drinks

# MICRONUTRIENTS

## Q145. What is Cholesterol?

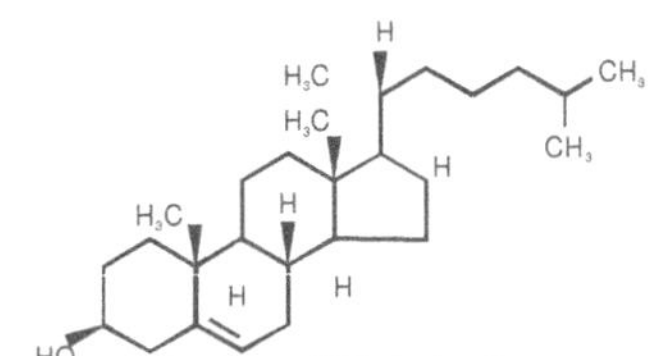


Structure of Cholesterol

**Ans** Cholesterol is a soft, waxy substance found among the lipids in the blood stream and in all body cells. It is normal to have cholesterol. It's an important part of a healthy body because it's used to form cell membranes some hormones and other needed tissues. But too high a level of cholesterol in the blood is a major risk for coronary heart disease, which leads to heart attack. It's also a risk factor for stroke. Hypercholesterolemia is the term for high levels of blood cholesterol. Body gets cholesterol in two ways. Body makes some of it and the rest comes from animal products that you eat, such as meat, poultry, fish, eggs, butter, cheese and whole milk. Food from plants like fruits, vegetables and cereals do not have cholesterol. SAAOL recommends removal of cholesterol from their patient's diet.

## Q146. What are foods that are high in Antioxidants?

**Ans** Foods that are high in antioxidants are red pepper, mangoes, avocado, broccoli, carrots, papaya, spinach etc. Without antioxidants, many of us would be prey to numerous infections. Although our bodies produce their own antioxidants, we also need to boost our defense by eating food that contain them. Antioxidants may also help to prevent premature ageing.

They protect against free radicals, which are formed in the body as part of its metabolism and defense against bacteria. To cope with these free radicals, the body needs more antioxidants than it can produce, particularly during times of illness or when exposed to pollutants. Fortunately, many foods provide antioxidants that help to protect the body against their threat.

Vitamin E, C and beta- carotene, the plant form of Vitamin A, help to neutralize free radicals, minerals such as selenium (found in avocados) and bio-flavonoid, found in some fruits and grapes also have antioxidant properties.

To obtain an adequate intake of antioxidants, it is safer to eat plenty of fresh fruit and vegetables. Citrus fruit provides Vitamin C and brightly colored fruit and vegetable supply beta- carotene.

### Q147. What are Fibres?

**Ans** Fibre is the material, which makes the cell wall in the plants and is the indigestible portion thereof. The body neither absorbs it nor the enzymes can break it down. It also helps in free movement of intestine and rules out inflammation and dryness of intestine, along with accumulated toxins.

Fibres are of two major kinds – soluble and insoluble. Certain vegetables and grain cereals have more insoluble fibre. Barley, oats, legumes and fruits contain more soluble fibre. Diet high in fiber and low in fat, yield soft, moist and plentiful stools and help in preventing and treating not only constipation but hemorrhoids also.

### Q148. How does Fibre help in reducing the chances of Heart Disease?

**Ans** Fibres are very useful component of our diet. They are of two types- soluble and insoluble. These two types of fibre bind the dietary cholesterol and does not allow it to get absorbed in the body. As we know cholesterol is known for creating blockages so, removal of cholesterol by fiber help in reducing the chances of heart disease.

## Q149 What are Vitamins?

**Ans** Organic substances in food are called Vitamins. They cannot be synthesized in enough quantities, even though they are required in small quantities. So far 13 vitamins, have been identified

### TABLE OF VITAMINS

Commonly used names

| | | | |
|---|---|---|---|
| 1. | Vitamin A | 8. | Folic acid |
| 2. | Thiamine | 9. | Vitamin B – 12 |
| 3. | Riboflavin | 10. | Vitamin C |
| 4. | Niacin | 11. | Vitamin D |
| 5. | Vitamin B – 6 | 12. | Vitamin E |
| 6. | Pantothenic Acid | 13. | Vitamin K |
| 7. | Biotin | | |

**VITAMIN – A (Retinol):-** Dietary sources of retinol are milk, Red fruits and yellow fruits, leafy vegetables which are of dark green colour. Carotene is found in carrots (they being the richest source).

**VITAMIN - C –**Vitamin C can be easily obtained from the dietary sources like oranges and various citrus fruits, guavas, black currants, green peppers, broccoli, raw cauliflower, sprouts of brussels, potatoes, cabbage, amla and lemon are still the largest

**Store houses of Vitamin C:-** It fastens healing process, holds all the cells of the body together, increases bodily resistance to fight infections and also forms a protective shield for defending the body from outside invasive forces. It also helps to build up resistance of entire body as a whole.

**VITAMIN – E (Tocopherol) –** It works as an antioxidant, protecting A, C and D Vitamins and also prevents fat from becoming rancid. It prevents formation of unwanted blood clots. It helps and promotes better blood circulation and promotes formation of healthy and new skin wounds. Oxygen and vitamin E are very important for each other. Its natural sources are wheat germ, leafy and green vegetables, and products of whole grains.

**Q150. If Minerals, Vitamins are zero calorie food than why do we need them?**

**Ans** The Vitamins mean "life substances" or "life elements". Vitamin a name derived from the Latin word "vita" meaning life and "amins" or amino acid, which are component parts of the protoplasm.

Vitamins are undoubtedly essential to life and are builders of our bodies. There are sixteen chemical elements of which the body is composed they are Oxygen, Nitrogen, Carbon, Chlorine, Fluorine, Phosphorus, Iron, Calcium, Potassium, Magnesium, Hydrogen, Sodium, Sulfur, Silica, Iodine and Manganese. Every element has to perform a special duty and if the blood and tissue building ones are not supplied in sufficient quantities or if any of them are missing, health will soon become impaired. Although the mineral elements make up only a comparatively small amount of the body say about 5 percent, they are nevertheless essential constituents and every single element has some distinct physiological function to perform. The normal and healthy development of the organism primarily depends upon the adequate supply of the organic salts, which truly may be called "the building stones of the body".

**Q151. How will you provide fat soluble vitamins in the body?Fat soluble vitamins are A, D, E, K**

**Ans.** :

1. **Vitamin A :** can be provided to the body in the form of carotene i.e. they are found in carrots, red fruits like pumpkin, melon, apricots and yellow fruits like leafy vegetables which are dark green.
2. **Vitamin D:** Its natural form, cholecalciferol is a modified steroid and is formed in the skin by the action of ultra violet light. Deficiency due to Vitamin D is liable to be felt due to lack of sunlight.
3. **Vitamin E:** It works as an antioxidant, protecting, A, C

and D. And also prevents fats from becoming rancid. Its natural sources are wheat germ, leafy and green vegetables and products of whole grains.

4. **Vitamin K:** It helps in maintaining clothing system in the blood. It can be obtained from wheat bran, wheat germ, cabbage, tomatoes, potatoes, spinach etc.

**Q152. How much calories one get on consumption of 1 gram of Vitamins and Minerals?**

**Ans** One gets ZERO CALORIES on consumption of 1 gram of vitamins and minerals.

**Q153. How does antioxidant help in preventing blockages in the heart?**

**Ans** Antioxidants are the nutrients which prevent oxidation of fat in the cells of the body. Vit. E or the tocopherol protects LDL or the bad cholesterol ( low density lipoproteins) from oxidation whereas Vit.C scanvenges free radicals and does not allow oxidationof the fat. When oxidation of the fat is prevented it does not settle in the blood artery, thus preventing blockages.

**Q154. What are the other important functions of Vitamin A,E,C?**

**Ans** The important functions of Vitamin A,E,C are:

Some Important Function of Vitamin A:

1. Eyesight particularly for night vision
2. Growth and tissue healing.
3. Healthy skin.
4. Antioxidant

Some Important functions of Vitamin C:

1. Formation of collagen, which is the biological cement that binds cells together in bones, teeth gums, blood vessels and connective tissue.

2. Aids in wound healing,
3. Helps in absorption of iron that forms your blood.
4. Acts as an antioxidant.
5. Regenerates oxidized vitamin E, helping it to returen to its active form.

**Some important functions of vitamin E:-**

1. An antioxidant that protects the unsaturated fatty acids located in the cell membrane and other body components from free radical attack.
2. It stimulates the immune response helping to build resistance to infection.
3. It inhibits the conversion of nitrities in smoked, pickled and cured foods to nitrosamines in the stomach.

## Q155. Is Water very essential for us?

**Ans** Most of us don't get enough of this precious stuff. As a result, we may look peaked and feel fatigued. Our bodies are composed of more fluid than anythingt else so water is a vital nutrient for our well- being.

**TIPS:**

1. Fill up a quart size water bottle and keep it with you for quick and refreshing drinks through out the day.
2. Don't rely on thirst ; this sensation diminishes with age. Drink often and choose from nutritious liquids, including 100% fruit and vegetable juices, skim or low fat milk, broths, sparkling water, and teas.
3. You can also get fluids from foods, especially those that are liquid at room temperature. Try gelatin, frozen yogurt, soups, water melon, pickles, oranges, lettuce, tomatoes etc.

# MACRONUTRIENT

**Q156. What are Carbohydrates?**

**Ans** Carbohydrates are composed of Carbon, Hydrogen and Oxygen in varying proportions supply energy for work, play and other forms of vital activity and furnish fuel to maintain heat. Carbohydrates are either simple or complex, and are the major source of energy in all human diets. They provide energy 4Kcal/g. The simple carbohydrates, glucose, and fructose are found if fruits, vegetables and honey, sucrose in sugar and lactose in milk and glycogen in animal foods. The other complex carbohydrates, which are resistant to digestion in human digestive tract are cellulose in vegetables, fruits and cereals, which constitute the dietary fiber component.

Dietary fibres delay and retard the absorption of carbohydrates and fats and increase satiety value. Diets rich in fiber reduce glucose and lipids in blood and increase the bulk of the stools. Diets rich in complex carbohydrates are healthier than low fiber diet based on the refined and processed foods.

**Q157. What is simple Carbohydrate?**

**Ans** When the basic glucose units are joined in a straight chain

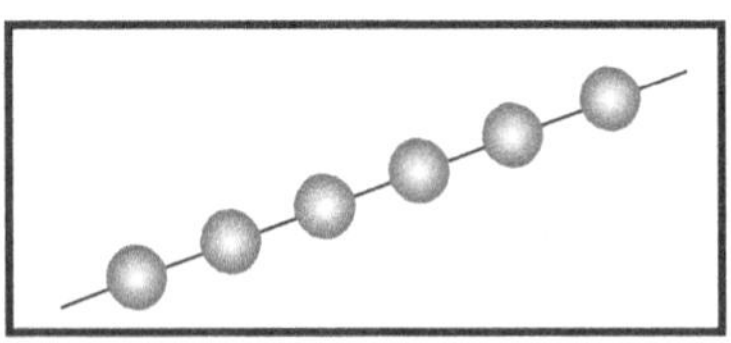

they are called as simple carbohydrates. As soon as they get into the digestive system the links break up very easily, which release glucose instantly, raising the blood glucose levels. Examples of these kinds of food is : Raw sugar, jaggery, sweets, candies, jam, jellies, cold drinks. Sweet fruits also fall in this group.

**Q158. What is complex Carbohydrate?**

**Ans** In these the glucose units are linked in a complex form i.e. branched structure. When this is put into the digestive system the links break up slowly, thus gradually releasing the glucose. So, there is a gradual increase in blood glucose levels. This allows insulin more time to work. examples are : Wheat rice, all cereals, brown bread, vegetables and fruits(non sweet).

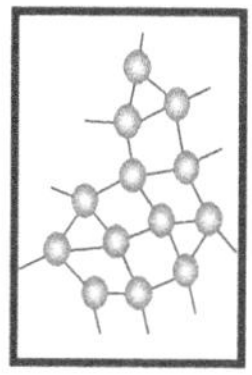

**Q159. What are Proteins?**

**Ans** Protein is composed of Carbon, Hydrogen, Oxygen and Nitrogen and is often termed as Nitrogenous foods. Protein is that element of the food, which is used for the construction and repair of the highly vitalized living tissues of the body; that is the essential vital machinery – the muscles, glands, nerves, and other parts concerned in the various functions of the body, consist of protein.

Protein is primary structural and functional component of every living cell. Almost half the protein in our body is in the form of muscles and rest of it is bone, cartilage and skin. Proteins are complex molecules composed of different amino acids. Certain amino acids have been termed as "essential" since they are not synthesized in the human body and have to be obtained from proteins in the diet. Other nonessential amino acids can be synthesized in the human body to build protein. Protein perform a wide range of functions and also provide energy (4 Kcal/g). Animal food like milk, meat, fish, eggs and plant foods such as legumes are rich source of protein. Animal protein is of high quality as it provides all the essential amino acids in right proportions. Plant or vegetable protein is not of the same quality because of their low content of some of the essential amino acids. However, a combination of cereals, millets and pulses provide most of the amino acids, which complement each other to provide the better quality of protein.

**Q160. What is the difference between Vegetarian and Non -Vegetarian protein?**

**Ans** There is a difference between vegetarian and non-vegetarian protein. We get vegetarian protein from plant sources and non- vegetarian protein from animal sources. Animal protein is of good quality as it provides all essential amino acids whereas plant protein lacks in one or the other essential amino acids. However, combination of various cereals and pulses will complement each other to provide better quality of protein.

**Q161. How much calorie one gets on consumption of 1gm of Carbohydrate?**

**Ans** 1gm of carbohydrate gives 4 calories.

**Q162. How much calorie is there in 1gm of protein?**

**Ans** 1gm of protein gives 4 calories.

**Q163. How much Calorie is there in 1 gm of fat?**

**Ans** 1gm of fat gives 9 calories.

# MODE OF COOKING

**Q164. Can heart patients make use of microwave cooking for preparing food?**

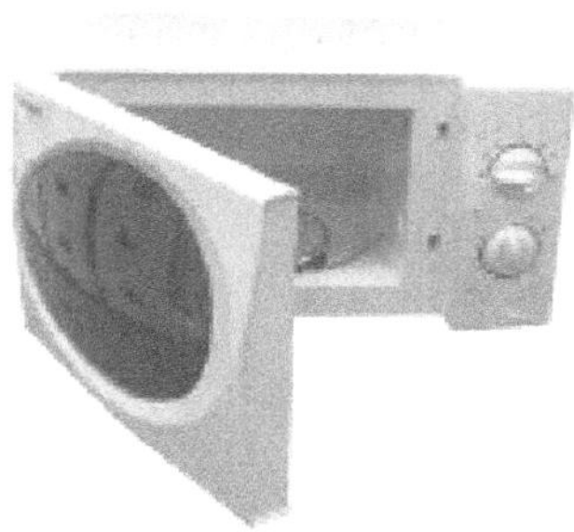

**Ans** Yes, heart patients can use microwave cooking. Microwave is a form of energy it is not heat. The principle of microwaves involve a type of electronic heating and is concerned with the production of high frequency waves from an oscillator tube called a magnetron. The electromagnetic waves have energy and this energy is transported to the desired load for heating. The energy created penetrates article of food to depth of "3" and causes the molecules that make up the food to rub together and create friction, supplying the heat, which cooks or reheats the food. Microwaves do not heat the oven cavity. Microwaves are reflected by many metal items and therefore are unsuitable for them. It is excellent as a re-heater.

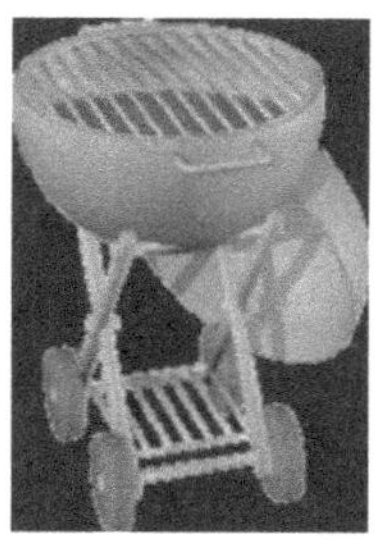

**Q165. Can one use grilling method for cooking food?**

**Ans** Yes, one can use grilling method for cooking food. Grilling consists of placing the food below or above a red-hot surface, when under the heater; the food is heated by radiation only.

This results in the browning of many food. Then the heat is more slowly conducted through the surfaces of the food downwards. As heating is mostly superficial, grilled food is usually reversed or rotated in the oven. If the food is above the heater heat is transmitted to the food through convection currents, as well as radiations with consequent increased efficiency.

Basic Rules of Grilling

1. Items for grilling must be small in size, flattened and on top
2. Heat should be intense to enable sealing at once and colouring a brown crust should form.
3. Grill bars should be cleaned.

**Q166. Can we make use of Roasting method?**

**Ans** Yes, you can make use of roasting method. Roasting is done by the direct exposure of the food to fire or on a hot vessel. Roasting involves no fat. Roasting is same as baking, but it is carried out in an oven temperature of $120^{\circ}$ to $126^{\circ}$ C. In roasting the food is partially cooked by dry heat and practically by moist heat, if the food has high moisture content. In roasting heat is transferred directly on to the container of the food through which it is conducted to the food.

**Q167. Can food be prepared by boiling?**

**Ans** Yes, food can be prepared by boiling. Boiling involves cooking in water. In this case the medium of transferring heat is water. Water receive heat by conduction through the sides of the utensils in which the food is cooked and pass on the heat by convection currents which equalizes the temperature and become very vigorous when boiling commences. Water is a poor conductor of heat and its heat capacity is high, i.e. it requires more heat than any other liquid of the same weight to raise the temperature. The boiling point of water is 100°C.

**Q168. Can we make use of Steaming?**

**Ans** Yes, you can make use of steaming method for cooking food. Steaming is cooking by moist heat, i.e. steam direct or indirect. Indirect steaming is done when the food is placed in a closed pan, which is surrounded by plenty of steam from fast boiling water or in a steamer. The food item could be protected with greaseproof paper or cloth or aluminum foil to prevent water getting into the food material.

Direct steaming is placing the article in a perforated container or on a covered plate over a source of water.

**Basic Rules:-**

1. Only suitable food items should be steamed, as it is cooked slowly. Green vegetables are not suitable as they loose Colour.
2. Root vegetables including potatoes must be placed on perforated tray, that will allow condensed steam to circulate and cook them.
3. It is a good method for invalids as the steamed foods are easily digested. Nourishment and flavour are retained in the food and usually the food cannot be easily over cooked.

**Q169. Can we make use of Baking?**

**Ans** Yes you can make use of baking. But in baking one should avoid greasing the baking tray. Baking is cooking of food by the action of dry heat in an oven. The degree of dryness of heat may be modified by the amount of steam produced from the items baked. Bread rolls, cakes, pastries, puddings, potatoes, vegetables, farinaceous dishes etc. are the products, which can be baked easily.

During baking the mixture or moisture in the product expands by air steam or carbon dioxide.

**Basic Rules**

Items should be placed in the right position in the oven; the cool spots should be avoided.

The oven should have the correct temperature according to the baked items, e.g. rich cake should have a lower temperature, than pastries, which should have a high temperature.

# MISCELLANEOUS

**Q170. Can I use Preservatives?**

**Ans** Yes, you can take food containing preservatives but it should not be in excess. Preservatives are basically chemicals. Some chemicals can prove hazardous to health such chemicals should be avoided. Commonly used preservative at home level are salt, oil, sugar syrup etc. such preservatives should be avoided by heart patients.

**Q171. Can I use colours in my food preparation?**

**Ans** Yes, you can use colours in your food preparation. So many synthetic and natural colours are being widely used in food items. Many of synthetic colors are potent carcinogenic and thus are restricted for use. But it is not possible to do away with synthetic colours completely. Though colours add nothing to the nutritive value of foods, it becomes necessary to restore the lost colour of the food during processing. Thus there is no harm in using colors, but better to use natural ones eg. Saffron, which is used for colouring has both flavouring and colouring properties.

**Q172. Can I put essence in my food?**

**Ans** Yes, you can put essence in your food. Essence is added in the food to give flavor and aroma. But some essences are made with certain oils such essence should be avoided.

**Q173. How to take Arjuna?**

**Ans** To prepare decoction, one teaspoon (5gm) of this powder should be boiled with one cup of water and reduced to one fourth.

This should be taken to cure heart diseases. Intake of this is also useful in bleeding dysentery and bleeding piles.

2. Milk preparation of Arjuna bark is an excellent remedy for all types of heart ailments. For its preparation, one tablespoon (15gm.) of coarse powder of this bark should be boiled in one cup of milk and four cups of water till one cup remains. This should be strained and given to the patient by adding sugar. It nourishes heart and heart muscles and cures different types of heart diseases. The powder of this bark and jaggery boiled in milk should be taken by a patient suffering from slow heart beat.

### Q174. What are the benefits of eating Arjuna?

**Ans** It is very useful in heart diseases and angina. It stimulates the heart, increases blood circulation, nourishes the heart muscles, regulates the heart beat and prevents the clotting in coronary arteries. It is also used in hamorrhages, leucorrhoea, dysentery, diarrhoea, fever, adiposity, liver disorder and sprue. It increases urine output. It is astringent and also used as a tonic and as an antidote to poison. It helps in healing the fractures of bones and ulcer.

### Q175. Should heart patients attend marriages?

**Ans** Yes, heart patients can attend marriages. Marriages are the occasions where you meet people and increase your acquaintance. Food should be secondary in such cases so, instead of thinking what to eat you should concentrate on guests and family members.

### Q176. What can we consume in the marriage parties?

**Ans** If one really wants to stick to regimen of eating zero oil foods one can still have plenty of choices in marriage parties too. In marriage parties there are always 2-3 varieties of salads. Then we have romali roti, tandoori roti, and boiled rice. One can have all this with curds or green chutneys. Have soup if you are sure enough that it is prepared without oil. Have fruit chaats, fruits juices if available.

**Q177. Can we eat in restaurant?**

**Ans** Eating in a restaurant is not a problem. You just have to make choice accordingly. If visiting a good restaurant then you can explain to the food in charge about the kind of zero oil food you want. Explain them the procedure to make zero oil food and they will try to provide the food you want because they are very particular about their prestige & reputation

**Q178. How one can order in north Indian restaurant?**

**Ans** It is not a difficult job to find and order zero oil food in a north Indian restaurant. In cereals one can ask for tandoori chapatti, romali roti, fried rice, dal without tarka, boiled potato with pieces. One can even guide a chef in the restaurant on how to prepare zero oil food. It is very easy to get vegetables like aloo methi, aloo chole, gobhi masala, stuffed baked brinjal etc. One can easily get curd, dhania pudina chutney or tomato chutney. In all one can order all these things:

Methi, Aloochole, Masala Gobhi with potatoes, Baigan Stuffed, Palak Paneer dal Urad Palak, Baigan Bharta, Masala band Gobhi, Masala Rajma Chole, Sarson da Sag, Kadhi, Masala Rice, Bhat Tomato, Makke di Roti, Nan, Cucumber Raita, Dahi Vadas, Pudina Raita, Black Carrot Pickle, Tomato Chutney Imli, Sprouted Moong salad.

**Q179. What one can order in south Indian restaurant?**

**Ans** Visiting south Indian restaurant and ordering zero oil food is very easy. Idli, Upma, Poha, Tomato bhat, even dosa and utpam all can be easily made without the use of single drop of oil. What it needs is a small interaction between the customer and chef or manager of the restaurant. Along with it you can order podi (roasted dal made into powder along with different spices) roasted dal chutney instead of coconut chutney, green chutney, tomato chutney, curd and even rasam & sambhar. Items of food which can be ordered are–

Plain Dosa, Buttermilk Dosa, Masala dosa, Rava Dosa, Bread Utppama, Shahi Vegetable Uppama, Idli, Masala Idli, Stuffed Idli, Vegetable Idli, Saga Idli, Sambhar Vada, Sagavada, Masala vada, Bonda, Dal Pakora.

**Q180. What one can order in Gujrati food?**

**Ans**
1. Khakra (Sada)
2. Bhat dhokli
3. Dhokla
4. Khandvi
5. Dhokla gavar
6. Crunchy potatoes
7. Aaloo poha
8. Palak Dal
9. Dal miloni
10. Raita Dhokla
11. Raita Baigan
12. Dal Thepla
13. Methi Bajari rotali
14. Bhakri Batata
15. Bhat borax
16. Lapsi

**Q181. What one can consume in Chinese food?**

**Ans** Sweet Corn Soup, Sizzling Soup, Green peas soup, Talomein Soup, Chinese Steamed Rice, Chilli Paneer, Cantonese vegetables, Chowmein.

**Q182. What kind of food one should eat while traveling in train?**

**Ans** There is vast variety of food items to choose when traveling. Any seasonal fruit like orange, apple, banana, guava, grapes, pears etc can be easily carried. In vegetables, salad vegetables can be taken along like carrot, radish, cucumber, boiled potatoes etc. In snacks one can choose from sandwiches, idli, Marie biscuits or Threptine biscuits, roasted chana, murmura, popcorns. In drinks you can have lemon water, if not diabetic then frooti, diet cold drinks, tea, coffee and if going for a short journey then one can very well prepare whole meal to take along-like chapatti or rice, dal without oil, any vegetable, green chutney, curd, any pickle made without oil. For e.g. Lemon pickle, carrot pickle etc.

**Q183. What kind of food one should eat while traveling in bus?**

**Ans** While traveling in a bus again one can easily carry any seasonal fruit or raw vegetables. Then other things like roasted chana, murmura, popcorns, Marie biscuits are there. If required carry soups like tomato soup or other vegetable soup in a flask. Take instant soup mixes with you, wherever at dhabas or restaurants you get hot water, mix the soup and your soup is ready.

**Q184. How to instruct waiters?**

**Ans** Ask them not to use oil for food. If possible explain them the process of frying without oil. Ask for chapattis without oil, rice without oil, salads. Ask for potato bharta or palak subji without oil. Give a good tip in advance.

**Q185. What kind of food one should eat while traveling in plane?**

**Ans** You can have variety of food in plane. Ask for things, which you are sure doesn't contain oil. Burger can be eaten but it should contain lot of filling (salads). Drinks like lemon juice, strawberry juice can be taken. Stuffed rotis with chutneys and sauces can be taken. Fruit salad, vegetable salad and sprout salad can be taken.

**Q186. What kind of food one can take while traveling by car on a long journey?**

Ans Food one can take while traveling by own car are as follows.

- Salads
- Any seasonal fruit like apple, papaya, litchi, guava.
- Any seasonal vegetable salad like cucumber, tomato, onion.
- Any pickle made without oil.
- Any chutney made without oil and coconut.
- Bread or pao.
- Home cooked food without oil.
- Instant soup mixes.
- Marie biscuits.

**Q187. What to order in roadside dhabas?**

Ans. In road side dhabas you can order the following things

- Salad
- Boiled dal without fried masala
- Boiled Potato
- Roti
- Rice

**Q188. Can I take Candies (Toffees without cream or milk)?**

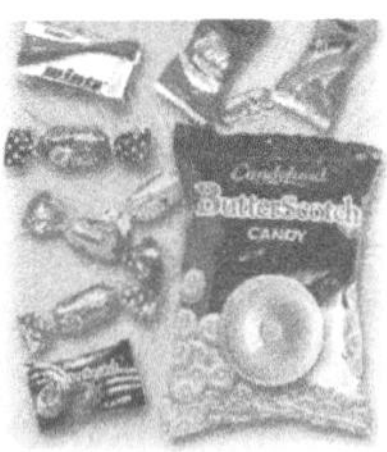


**Ans** Yes, you can take candies. Most of them are made of sugar or sweeteners and do not have any oil items. If you are not a diabetic you can consume candies. These candies have artificial colours, which are not contra-indicated for heart patients.

**Q189. Can I take Chocolate?**

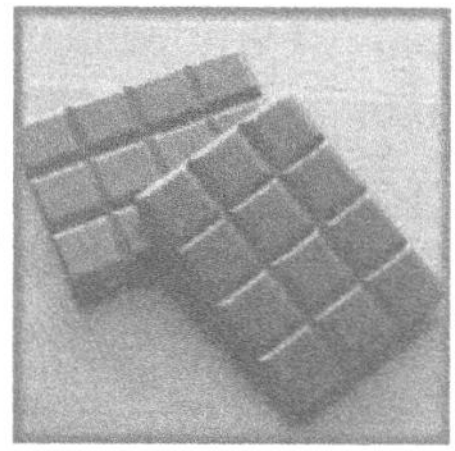

**Ans** Nutritionally Chocolate contains some protein, variable amounts of sugar and certain minerals. Plain chocolate is a useful source of iron and magnesium, for example and all chocolate contains potassium. Chocolate also contains compounds, which act as mild stimulants, which may also be responsible for causing migrane.

Chocolate is high in fat- about 30% by weight – it is also high in calorie, containing around 500 calories per 100 grams. Chocolate also contain the stimulants theobromine and caffeine.

Adding sugar, additional fat and milk makes chocolate confectionery. The fat added to chocolate is cocoa butter, which gives the characteristic melt in mouth texture. Chocolate contains five percent vegetable fat so it is to be avoided by heart patients as it increases the blood Triglyceride level.

**Q190. Can I take Lauki juice?**

**Ans** Yes, you can take Lauki juice if you want as it helps to lower Cholesterol. Also it is beneficial for loosing extra weight.

**Q191. Is Gelatin be used?**

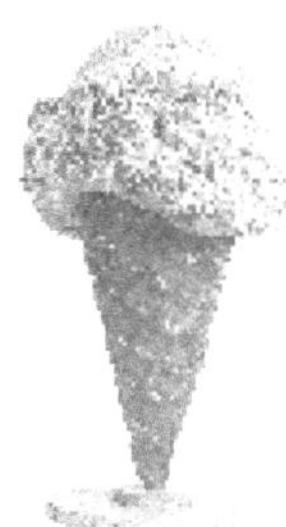

**Ans** No, Gelatin cannot be used, as it is bone tendons and ligaments containing collagen, which by hydrolysis when treated by boiling water is transformed into gel. Gelatin is a protein food but is used in diet chiefly for its mechanical effect. As it is from animal source it should be avoided.

**Q192. Can I eat Ice cream?**

**Ans** Yes, you can have ice cream but it should be home made i.e. made up of skimmed milk by adding custard powder, corn flour, china grass, breadcrumbs as a thickening agent but while having the home made ice cream your milk intake i.e., 200 ml has to be adjusted for the whole day.

If you want to have ice cream from the market then you can have candies i.e. ice balls.

**Q193. What kind of Salad dressings can be used?**

**Ans** Salad dressings without oil should be used. In such dressings vinegar is used as a base.

**Q194. What to do if I have constipation?**

**Ans** Some home Remedies for short-term relief from constipation are

1. Take 'Isabgol' powder or 'Nature Care' (Dabur) with hot milk/hot water at night.
2. Take 'Trifla' or 'Harar' or 'Amla' powder with hot milk / hot water at night.
3. Take hot water mixed with salt just after getting up in the morning and walk for few minutes before going for clearing bowels.
4. Take honey and lemon in hot water in morning after getting up.
5. Take prunes (Moonakka) after boiling in milk.
6. Take 'Gulkand' with hot milk at night.
7. Take some Ayurvedic formulations for bowel evacuations with water at night.
8. Take castor oil at night
9. Cut a lemon into two halves. Apply some salt and black pepper on it and directly suck its juice in the mouth, finish one full lemon.
10. Take 'enema' of lukewarm water in which some salt or lemon can be mixed.
11. One should drink six to eight glasses of water each day.
12. Taking a high fiber and roughage diet e.g. whole grain

cereals and pulses, leafy vegetables like spinach, raw carrots, reddish, cucumber, salad, fruits like prunes, figs, papaya, oranges, water melon and other fresh fruits. Avoid refined and processed food and food with no fiber e.g. white flour 'Maida', white sugar and their preparations

13. Take green Colour water. This water is prepared by keeping water in a green colour glass bottle in sunshine for about 8 hrs. By this, water absorbs the green colour from sunrays and this colour is good for removing constipation.
14. Sit in Vajrasana off and on and specially after eating food. Vajrasana increases the circulation in the abdomen and there by increases the tone and efficiency of large intestines.
15. Consume eatables having lot of potassium e.g. banana, potato, tomato etc.

**Q195. Can heart patients take Yeast?**

**Ans** Yes, Yeast is another form of ready made leavening agent for processing of bread and other bakery products. An elderly person, who still uses yeast tablets for upkeep of his health and even after being above 90 years age, is mentally and physically hale, hearty and fit. Leavened food not only arouses digestive faculties but is also effective in cancer and arthritis, in toning up nervous system. Its taste is sour and is easily digested.

**Q196. How can I know that how much calorie is present in my food?**

**Ans** It is very simple to count your calories. First and foremost you should know how much calorie does carbohydrate, fat and protein give. 1gm of carbohydrate gives 4 calories, 1gm of fat gives 9 calories and 1gm of protein gives 4 calories. Now you should know whether food is a carbohydrate source or fat source or protein source. After this weigh your food item and multiply by the given calorie of the source eg. Suppose you have bread slice which weighs 25gms excluding water. Now multiply 25gms with four, as it is a carbohydrate source. So you get 100 calories. Like this you can count calories in your food.

**Q197. Can silver paper be used for decoration**

**Ans** Yes, silver paper can be used for decoration. Silver is a mineral like iron, calcium etc. which is needed by our body in very little quantity. You can make use of this mineral in your diet through decoration foils. Now a days diabetes is known to be treated with these minerals (silver, gold etc.)

**Q198. Can I take B-complex supplement?How will they be helpful?**

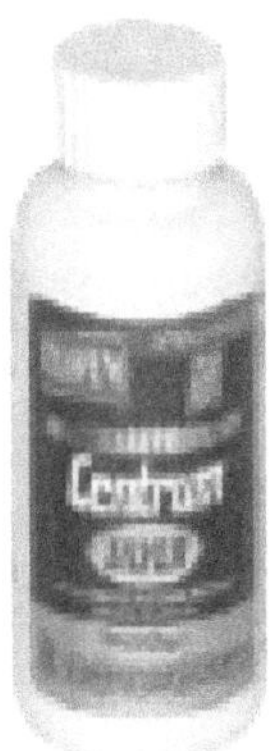

**Ans** Yes, you can take B- complex supplements. In the present world our diet is not fully equipped with nutrients that is why we are suffering from so many diseases. One of the main reasons for such problems is the reduction in B-complex vitamins. These vitamins help in resurrection of our intestinal microflora, which is helpful in our digestion and absorption. These vitamins also help in preventing various diseases like heart diseases, cancer and intestinal disorderd etc.

**Q199. Can I take health drinks like Milo, Bournvita etc.?**

**Ans** No, you should avoid health drinks. Health drinks are good ready made supplement of nutrients. But before taking health drinks you should know about its composition, specially you should know about its fat content.If that is more then you should avoid such drinks.In India they do not write about the exact food content but most of these drinks have high Milk fat/Milk solids. Apart from this diabetic heart patients should avoid these drinks because it contains simple sugar which raise the blood sugar.

**Q.200 What can you eat if you have diabetes and acid reflux?**

**Ans** If you follow the following advice it might help you to get better.

**Step 1** Eat frequent, small meals instead of less-frequent big meals.(This is also a helpful eating style for people with type 2 diabetes.)

**Step 2** Lose some extra weight if you are overweight, but not by fad dieting. (This is also a crucial step for people who are overweight and have type 2 diabetes.)

**Step 3** Avoid eating high-fat meals when possible to encourage weight loss (if appropriate) and to reduced acid reflux.

**Step 4** Avoid fried or fatty food

The following drinks encourage acid reflux and should be limited, particularly before bed:

- Coffee
- Caffeinated tea
- Cola drinks
- Alcoholic beverages

Step 5 Food that increase the acid content of the stomach should be consumed in small portions or limited quantity.

- Coffee
- Caffeinated tea and cola

Calcium in milk (It has been suggested that the calcium in milk increases stomach acid secretion).

**Step 6** Food that irritate a damaged esophageal lining should be limited (if your lining is damaged):

- Citrus fruits

- Tomatoes and tomato products
- Pepper
- Chilli pepper

**Step 7** Food that bloat the abdomen, causing pressure that forces acid to back up into the esophagus, should be limited.

- All carbonated beverages

**Step 8** Have your heartburn helpers handy.

- Antacids or lozenges

Chewing gum that isn't flavored with peppermint or spearming

(Just make sure it's sugar free gum so you aren't added sugar this way.)

- Plain old tap water

(Drinking plenty of water is good for people with diabetes too- you want to keep the kidneys as healthy as possible since people with diabetes are at an increased risk of kidney failure.)

Eating sweet pickles has been suggested by some to help with reflux.

**Step 9** Don't eat three to four hours before going to bed.

(Some people with diabetes need to plan a late-night snack as part of keeping their blood sugars normal, but others do better without a late-night snack as a way of cutting overall calories in an attempt to lose weight to improve their diabetes.)

**Step 10** Make other lifestyle changes that can help your heartburn, such as quitting smoking and elevating the head of your bed 6 inches.

(No smoking is also helpful for those with diabetes as a way of reducing the risk of heart disease, which they are at increased risk for.)

**Q 201 Is reversal diet appropriate for heart patients needing to gain weight?**

**Ans** People who follow reversal diet and lifestyle recommendations lose weight if they are over weight, but their weight tends to plateau when they reach a weight that's right for them. If the food tastes good, and if they can get help with their underlying depression (assuming that this is a factor), then they should be able to maintain or gain weight as needed. When they loose wight we can give them Zero oil high calorie food to arrest the weight loss and even can increase weight.

# A QUICK GUIDE TO FATS

Fat or oil (lipid is the biochemical term) is one of the six basic food groups. Fats and oils are made of building blocks called fatty acids. Structurally, a fatty acid is a chain of carbon atoms with a certain quantity of hydrogen atoms attached; the more hydrogen atoms attached, the more "saturated" the fat. Fats come in three natural forms (called hydrogenated or trans fats).

**Saturated Fats-** Saturated fats are solid at room temperature and are primarily found in animal food and tropical oil, such as coconut and palm oil. A fatty acid that has its full quota of hydrogen atoms is a saturated fatty acid. The body produces saturated fats from sugar, which is one reason why low-fat food do not decrease body fat-their high sugar content is converted into stored fat in the body. Although high fat intake from animal sources have been associated with heart disease, some amount of saturated fat in the diet is necessary to help the body's cells remain healthy and resistant to disease.

**Unsaturated Fats-** Unsaturated fatty acids (both monounsaturated and polyunsaturated) are liquid at room temperature. Most vegetable oils are unsaturated. Unsaturated means some of the carbon molecules are not filled with hydrogen.

**Monounsaturated Fats:** When a fatty acid lacks only two hydrogen atoms, it is a monounsaturated fatty acid. Monounsaturated fats are considered healthier than polyunsaturated fats because of their ability to lower blood levels of bad cholesterol and maintain or raise levels of good cholesterol. Canola oil and olive oil are naturally high in monounsaturated fats. Olive oil is the best oil for cooking, because it does not break down easily into singlet oxygen molecules (free radicals) like most oils do when they are heated. Olive oil is probably the most widely used oil, both for cooking and raw on salads, on a worldwide basis.

**Polyunsaturated Fats:** Oils high in polyunsaturated fats include flaxseed and canola oils, as well as pumpkin seeds, purslane, hemp oil, walnuts, and soybeans, which contain omega-3 and omega-6 essential fatty acids. A fatty acid lacking four or more hydrogen atoms is a polyunsaturated fatty acid. They can be found in both healthy and unhealthy fats and oils.

**Hydrogenated and Trans Fats-** These terms refer to a synthetic process in which natural oils are broken down into a semi-solid fat by adding a hydrogen atom to an unsaturated fat molecule. This process is widely used to prolong the shelf life of commercial baked goods, packaged foods, most salad oils and dressings, margarine, and cooking oils. The molecules that make up these fats, called trans-fatty acids, are known to interfere with the healthy functioning of our bodies due to their unusual molecular shape.

**Essential Fatty Acids(EFAs)-** Unsaturated fats required in the diet are called essential fatty acids. Omega-3 and omega-6 oils are the two principle types of EFAs and a balance of these oils in the diet is necessary for good health. The primary omega-3 oil is alpha-linolenic acid (ALA), found in flaxseed and canola oils, as well as pumpkin seeds, walnuts, and soybeans. Fish oils, as well as pumpkin seeds, walnuts, and soyabeans. Fish oils, such as salmon, cod, and mackerel, contain the other important omega-3 oils, DHA (docosahexaenoic acid) and EPA (eicosapentaenoic acid). Linoleic acid is the main omega-6 oil and is found in most vegetable oils, including safflower, corn, peanut, and seasame. The most therapeutic form of omega-6 oil is gamma-linolenic acid (GLA), found in evening primrose, black currant, and borage oils. Once in the body, omega-3 and omega-6 are converted to prostaglandins, hormone-like complex fatty acids that affect smooth muscle function, inflammatory processes, and constriction and dilation of blood vessels.

# ANTIOXIDANT PROTECTION

An antioxidant is a natural biochemical substance that protects living cells from the damaging effects of free radicals. Free radicals cause oxidation, the same chemical process that causes metal to rust and apples to turn brown. In the body, if left uncontrolled, free radicals cause cell membranes to erode and die, leading to a variety of degenerative conditions.

Produced as a by-product of cellular activities, free radicals are typically neutralized and rendered harmless by antioxidants. But when environmental and other toxins (poor diet, pollution, stress, cigarettes) introduce an increased burben of free radicals, the body's reserve of antioxidants is quickly exhausted.

**Types of Antioxidants-**

- ***Amino Acids:*** cysteine, glutathione, methionine
- ***Bioflavonoids:*** anthocyanin bioflavonoids (in fruit, especially grapes, cranberries, and bilberries), citrus bioflavonoids (in grapefruit, lemons, and oranges), oligometric proanthocyanidins (OPCs) in pycnogenol (pine bark or grape seed extract)
- ***Carotene:*** alpha and beta carotene (in red, yellow, and dark green fruits and vegetables) Lycopene (in red fruits and vegetables, such as red grapefruit and tomatoes
- ***Spices:*** cayenne pepper, garlic, turmeric
- ***Herbs:*** astragalus, bilberry, ginkgo, green tea, milk thistle, saga

- ***Minerals:*** copper, maganese, selenium, zinc
- ***Vitamins:*** A, B1, C and E coenzyme Q10, NADH (nicotinamide adenine dinucleotide)
- ***Enzymes:*** catalase, glutathione peroxidase, superoxide dismutase
- ***Hormones:*** melatonin
- ***Miscellaneous:*** lipoid acid.

# FOOD ITEMS TO BE AVOIDED

1. Milk (full cream) and Milk Products
2. Skimmed Milk (*Bina vasa ka Doodh*) - beyond 200 ml per day
3. Cheese and Butter
4. Butter Milk (*Lassi*) beyond 200 ml of milk (skimmed)
5. All kinds of Non-vegetarian items
6. Nuts and Dry fruits
7. Sweets (*Mithai*) which contain fat and oil
8. Oil (All types of oils).

# FOOD ITEMS MODERATELY RESTRICTED

1. Brown Bread and White Bread (Double Roti)
2. Rice (Chawal)
3. Vermicelli (Sewai)
4. Bajra (Bajra)
5. Jowar
6. Maize (Makka)
7. Chapati, Roti, Phulka (Wheat)
8. Peas (Dry) (Matar Sukha)
9. Potato, Sweet Potato (Shakarkandi), Arvi
10. Jaggery (Gur), Sugar (Chini)
11. Cane Sugar (Chini)
12. Banana (Ripe) (Kela)
13. Mango
14. Cold Drinks
15. Thick Dal

# FOOD ITEMS WHICH CAN BE CONSUMED FREELY

**Cereals**

1. Rice puffed (Murmura)
2. Rice, flakes (Chiwra Poha)

**Pulses**

3. Bengal Gram (Whole), (Chana)
4. Bengal Gram, Dal (Chana Ki Dal)
5. Bengal Gram, roasted (Bhuna Chana)
6. Black Gram, Dal (Urad Dal)
7. Cow Pea (Lobia)
8. Green Gram, whole (Moong)
9. Green Gram Dal (Moong ki Dal)
10. Horse Gram, whole (Kulthi)
11. Lentil (Masoor Tur)
12. Moth Beans (Moth)
13. Green Peas (Matar)
14. Rajmah (Rajmah)
15. Red Gram, Dal (Arhal Dal)
16. Soyabean (Bhatmas)

**Leafy Vegetables**

17. Bathua Leaves (Bathua Sag)

18. Spinach (Palak)
19. Radish Leaves (Mooli ka Saag)
20. Cabbage (Patta Gobhi)
21. Amaranth (Cholai Saag)
22. Carrot Leaves (Gajar Saag)
23. Radish Leaves (Muli ka Saag)
24. Calocasia Leaves (Arvi ka Saag)
25. Drumstick (Saijan)
26. Fenugreek (Methi Saag)
27. Lettuce (Salad leaves)
28. Mint (Pudina)
29. Mustard Leaves (Sarson Saag)

**Roots and Tubers**

30. Yam, ordinary (Jimikand)
31. Carrot (Gajar)
32. Onion (Pyaj)
33. White Radish (Safed Mooli)
34. Garlic
35. Ginger

**Other Vegetables**

36. Beans (Sem)
37. Brinjal (Baigan)
38. Cucumber (Khira Kakdi)
39. French Beans
40. Lotus stem (Dry) (Kamal Gatta)
41. Parwar (Parwal)
42. Pumpkin (Kaddu)

43. Lady-finger (Bhindi)
44. Tinda (Tinda)
45. Tomato (Tamatar)
46. Bottle Gourd (Ghia)
47. Turai
58. Cucumber (Kheera)
49. Capsicum (Shimla Mirch)
50. Kakri
51. Mushrooms

**Fruits**

52. Apple (Seb)
53. Guava (Amrood)
54. Lemon (Nimbu)
55. Sweet Lime (Mousomi)
56. Orange (Santara)
57. Water Melon (Tarbooj)
58. Papaya (Ripe) (Papita)
59. Pineapple (Ananas)
60. Tomato Ripe
61. Musk Melon (Kharbooza)

# Nutrient Value of Indian Foods

*(All the values are per 100 g of edible portion)*

| Food Stuff | Moisture (g) | Protein (g) | Fat (g) | Carbohydrate (g) | Fibre (g) | Energy (Cal) |
|---|---|---|---|---|---|---|
| **Cereals** | | | | | | |
| 1. Bajra | 12.4 | 11.6 | 5.0 | 67.5 | 1.2 | 361 |
| 2. Barley (jau) | 12.5 | 11.5 | 1.3 | 69.6 | 3.9 | 336 |
| 3. Jowar | 11.9 | 10.4 | 1.9 | 72.6 | 1.6 | 349 |
| 4. Maize (makai) | 14.9 | 11.1 | 3.6 | 66.2 | 2.7 | 342 |
| 5. Rice | 13.7 | 6.8 | 0.5 | 78.2 | 0.2 | 345 |
| 6. Rice flakes | 12.2 | 6.6 | 1.2 | 77.3 | 0.7 | 346 |
| 7. Rice puffed | 14.7 | 7.5 | 0.1 | 73.6 | 0.3 | 325 |
| 8. Wheat, whole | 12.8 | 12.1 | 1.7 | 69.4 | 1.9 | 341 |
| 9. Wheat flour | 12.2 | 12.1 | 1.7 | 69.4 | 1.9 | 341 |
| 10. Refined flour | 13.3 | 11.0 | 0.9 | 73.9 | 0.3 | 348 |

| | Food Stuff | Moisture (g) | Protein (g) | Fat (g) | Carbohydrate (g) | Fibre (g) | Energy (Cal) |
|---|---|---|---|---|---|---|---|
| 11. | Semolina (suji) | – | 10.4 | 0.8 | 74.8 | 0.2 | 348 |
| 12. | Vermicelli | 11.7 | 8.7 | 0.4 | 78.3 | 0.2 | 352 |
| 13. | Brown bread | 39.0 | 8.8 | 1.4 | 49.0 | 1.2 | 244 |
| 14. | White bread | 39.0 | 7.8 | 0.7 | 51.9 | 0.2 | 245 |
| **Pulses** | | | | | | | |
| 15. | Bengal gram whole | 9.8 | 17.1 | 5.3 | 60.9 | 3.9 | 360 |
| 16. | Bengal gram dal | 9.9 | 20.8 | 5.6 | 59.8 | 1.2 | 372 |
| 17. | Roasted Bengal gram | 10.7 | 22.5 | 5.2 | 58.1 | 1.0 | 369 |
| 18. | Black gram dal | 10.9 | 24.0 | 1.4 | 59.6 | 0.9 | 347 |
| 19. | Cowpea (Lobia) | 13.4 | 24.1 | 1.0 | 54.5 | 3.8 | 323 |
| 20. | Green gram (whole) | 10.4 | 24.0 | 1.3 | 56.7 | 4.1 | 334 |
| 21. | Green gram (dal) | 10.1 | 24.5 | 1.2 | 59.9 | 0.8 | 348 |
| 22. | Lentil | 12.4 | 25.1 | 0.7 | 59.0 | 0.7 | 343 |
| 23. | Moth beans | 10.8 | 23.6 | 1.1 | 56.6 | 4.5 | 330 |

| Food Stuff | Moisture (g) | Protein (g) | Fat (g) | Carbohydrate (g) | Fibre (g) | Energy (Cal) |
|---|---|---|---|---|---|---|
| 24. Peas (dry) | 16.0 | 19.7 | 1.1 | 56.5 | 4.5 | 315 |
| 25. Rajmah | 12.0 | 22.9 | 1.3 | 60.6 | 4.8 | 346 |
| 26. Redgram dal | 13.4 | 22.3 | 1.7 | 57.6 | 1.5 | 335 |
| 27. Soyabean | 8.1 | 43.2 | 19.5 | 20.9 | 3.7 | 432 |
| **Leafy Vegetables** | | | | | | |
| 28. Bathua | 89.6 | 3.7 | 0.4 | 2.9 | 0.8 | 30 |
| 29. Beet greens | 86.4 | 3.4 | 0.8 | 6.5 | 0.7 | 46 |
| 30. Brussel sprouts | 85.5 | 4.7 | 0.5 | 7.1 | 1.2 | 52 |
| 31. Cabbage | 91.9 | 1.8 | 0.1 | 4.6 | 1.0 | 27 |
| 32. Carrot leaves | 76.6 | 5.1 | 0.5 | 13.1 | 1.9 | 77 |
| 33. Colocasia leaves | 82.7 | 3.9 | 1.5 | 6.8 | 2.9 | 36 |
| 34. Coriander leaves | 86.3 | 3.3 | 0.6 | 6.3 | 1.2 | 44 |
| 35. Curry leaves | 63.8 | 6.1 | 1.0 | 18.7 | 6.4 | 108 |
| 36. Fenugreek leaves | 86.1 | 4.4 | 0.9 | 6.0 | 1.1 | 49 |

| Food Stuff | Moisture (g) | Protein (g) | Fat (g) | Carbohydrate (g) | Fibre (g) | Energy (Cal) |
|---|---|---|---|---|---|---|
| 37. Lettuce | 93.4 | 2.1 | 0.3 | 2.5 | 0.5 | 21 |
| 38. Mint | 84.9 | 4.8 | 0.6 | 5.8 | 2.0 | 48 |
| 39. Mustard leaves | 89.8 | 4.0 | 0.6 | 3.2 | 0.8 | 34 |
| 40. Radish leaves | 90.8 | 3.8 | 0.4 | 2.4 | 1.0 | 28 |
| 41. Spinach | 92.1 | 2.0 | 0.7 | 2.9 | 0.6 | 26 |
| **Roots and Tubers** | | | | | | |
| 42. Beet root | 87.1 | 1.7 | 0.1 | 8.8 | 0.9 | 43 |
| 43. Carrot | 86.0 | 0.9 | 0.2 | 10.6 | 1.2 | 48 |
| 44. Colocasia | 73.1 | 3.0 | 0.1 | 21.1 | 1.0 | 97 |
| 45. Onion | 84.3 | 1.8 | 0.1 | 12.6 | 0.6 | 59 |
| 46. Potato | 74.7 | 1.6 | 0.1 | 22.6 | 0.4 | 97 |
| 47. Radish | 94.4 | 0.7 | 0.1 | 3.4 | 0.8 | 17 |
| 48. Sweet potato | 68.5 | 1.2 | 0.3 | 28.2 | 0.8 | 120 |
| 49. Tapioca | 59.4 | 0.7 | 0.2 | 38.1 | 0.6 | 157 |
| 50. Turnip | 91.6 | 0.5 | 0.2 | 6.2 | 0.9 | 29 |

| Food Stuff | | Moisture (g) | Protein (g) | Fat (g) | Carbohydrate (g) | Fibre (g) | Energy (Cal) |
|---|---|---|---|---|---|---|---|
| **Other Vegetables** | | | | | | | |
| 51. | Bitter gourd | 92.4 | 1.6 | 0.2 | 4.2 | 0.8 | 25 |
| 52. | Bottle gourd | 96.1 | 0.2 | 0.1 | 2.5 | 0.6 | 12 |
| 53. | Brinjal | 92.7 | 1.4 | 0.3 | 4.0 | 1.3 | 24 |
| 54. | Broad beans | 85.4 | 4.5 | 0.1 | 7.2 | 2.0 | 48 |
| 55. | Cauliflower | 90.8 | 2.6 | 0.4 | 4.0 | 1.2 | 30 |
| 56. | Cucumber | 96.3 | 0.4 | 0.1 | 2.5 | 0.4 | 13 |
| 57. | Drumstick | 86.9 | 2.5 | 0.1 | 3.7 | 4.8 | 26 |
| 58. | French beans | 91.4 | 1.7 | 0.1 | 4.5 | 1.8 | 26 |
| 59. | Capsicum | 92.4 | 1.3 | 0.3 | 4.3 | 1.0 | 24 |
| 60. | Jack tender (kathal) | 84.0 | 2.6 | 0.3 | 9.4 | 2.8 | 51 |
| 61. | Ladies fingers | 89.6 | 1.9 | 0.2 | 6.4 | 1.2 | 35 |
| 62. | Lotus stem (dry) | 9.5 | 4.1 | 1.3 | 51.4 | 25.0 | 234 |
| 63. | Mango (green) | 87.5 | 0.7 | 0.1 | 10.1 | 1.2 | 44 |
| 64. | Onion stalks | 87.6 | 0.1 | 0.2 | 8.9 | 1.6 | 41 |
| 65. | Parwar | 92.0 | 2.0 | 0.3 | 2.2 | 3.0 | 20 |

| Food Stuff | Moisture (g) | Protein (g) | Fat (g) | Carbohydrate (g) | Fibre (g) | Energy ((Cal) |
|---|---|---|---|---|---|---|
| 66. Plantain (green) | 83.2 | 1.4 | 0.2 | 14.0 | 0.7 | 64 |
| 67. Pumpkin | 92.6 | 1.4 | 0.1 | 4.6 | 0.7 | 25 |
| 68. Ridge gourd | 95.2 | 0.5 | 0.1 | 3.4 | 0.5 | 17 |
| 69. Tinda | 93.5 | 1.4 | 0.2 | 3.4 | 1.0 | 21 |
| 70. Tomato (green) | 93.1 | 1.9 | 0.1 | 3.6 | 0.7 | 23 |
| 71. Water chestnut | 70.0 | 4.7 | 0.3 | 23.3 | 0.6 | 115 |
| **Nuts and Oilseeds** | | | | | | |
| 72. Almond | 5.2 | 20.8 | 58.9 | 10.5 | 1.7 | 655 |
| 73. Arecanut (supari) | 31.3 | 4.9 | 4.4 | 47.2 | 11.2 | 249 |
| 74. Cashewnut | 5.9 | 21.2 | 46.9 | 22.3 | 1.3 | 596 |
| 75. Chilgoza | 4.0 | 13.9 | 49.3 | 29.0 | 1.0 | 615 |
| 76. Coconut (dry) | 4.3 | 6.8 | 62.3 | 18.4 | 66.6 | 662 |
| 77. Coconut (fresh) | 36.3 | 4.5 | 41.6 | 13.0 | 3.6 | 444 |
| 78. Coconut (tender) | 90.8 | 0.9 | 1.4 | 6.3 | – | 41 |
| 79. Coconut (milk) | 42.8 | 3.4 | 41.0 | 11.9 | – | 430 |

| Food Stuff | Moisture (g) | Protein (g) | Fat (g) | Carbohydrate (g) | Fibre (g) | Energy (Cal) |
|---|---|---|---|---|---|---|
| 80. Coconut (water) | 93.8 | 1.4 | 0.1 | 4.4 | - | 24 |
| 81. Gingelly seeds (til) | 5.3 | 18.3 | 43.3 | 25.0 | 2.9 | 563 |
| 82. Groundnut | 3.0 | 25.3 | 40.1 | 26.1 | 3.1 | 567 |
| 83. Groundnut (roasted) | 1.7 | 26.2 | 39.8 | 26.7 | 3.1 | 570 |
| 84. Mustard seeds | 8.5 | 20.0 | 39.7 | 23.8 | 1.8 | 541 |
| 85. Pistachio nut | 5.6 | 19.8 | 53.5 | 16.2 | 2.1 | 626 |
| 86. Piyal seeds (chironji) | 3.0 | 19.0 | 59.1 | 12.1 | 3.8 | 656 |
| 87. Walnut | 4.5 | 15.6 | 64.5 | 11.0 | 2.6 | 687 |
| **Spices** | | | | | | |
| 88. Asafetida (Hing) | 16.0 | 4.0 | 1.1 | 67.8 | 4.1 | 297 |
| 89. Cardamom | 20.0 | 10.2 | 2.2 | 42.1 | 20.1 | 229 |
| 90. Chillies (dry) | 10.0 | 15.9 | 6.2 | 31.6 | 30.2 | 246 |
| 91. Chillies (green) | 85.7 | 2.9 | 0.6 | 3.0 | 6.8 | 29 |
| 92. Cloves | 25.2 | 5.2 | 8.9 | 46.0 | 9.5 | 286 |
| 93. Coriander | 11.2 | 14.1 | 16.1 | 21.6 | 32.6 | 288 |

| Food Stuff | Moisture (g) | Protein (g) | Fat (g) | Carbohydrate (g) | Fibre (g) | Energy (Cal) |
|---|---|---|---|---|---|---|
| 94. Cumin seeds | 11.9 | 18.7 | 15.0 | 36.6 | 12.0 | 356 |
| 95. Fenugreek seeds | 13.7 | 26.2 | 5.8 | 44.1 | 7.2 | 333 |
| 96. Garlic | 62.0 | 6.3 | 0.1 | 29.8 | 0.8 | 145 |
| 97. Ginger | 80.9 | 2.3 | 0.9 | 12.3 | 2.4 | 67 |
| 98. Mango powder (amchoor) | 6.8 | 2.8 | 7.8 | 64.0 | 13.7 | 337 |
| 99. Black pepper | 18.2 | 11.5 | 6.8 | 49.2 | 14.9 | 304 |
| 100. Poppy seeds (postdana) | 4.3 | 21.7 | 19.3 | 36.8 | 8.0 | 408 |
| 101. Tamarind pulp | 20.9 | 3.1 | 0.1 | 67.4 | 5.6 | 283 |
| 102. Turmeric | 1331 | 6.3 | 5.1 | 69.4 | 2.6 | 349 |
| **Fruits** | | | | | | |
| 103. Amla | 81.8 | 0.5 | 0.1 | 13.7 | 3.4 | 58 |
| 104. Apple | 84.6 | 0.2 | 0.5 | 13.4 | 1.0 | 59 |
| 105. Apricot, fresh | 85.3 | 1.0 | 0.3 | 11.6 | 1.1 | 53 |

| Food Stuff | Moisture (g) | Protein (g) | Fat (g) | Carbohydrate (g) | Fibre (g) | Energy (Cal) |
|---|---|---|---|---|---|---|
| 106. Apricot, dry | 19.4 | 1.6 | 0.7 | 73.4 | 2.1 | 306 |
| 107. Ball fruit | 61.5 | 1.8 | 0.3 | 31.8 | 2.9 | 137 |
| 108. Banana | 70.1 | 1.2 | 0.3 | 21.2 | 0.4 | 116 |
| 109. Cape gooseberry (Raspberry) | 82.9 | 1.8 | 0.2 | 11.1 | 3.2 | 53 |
| 110. Red cherries | 83.4 | 1.1 | 0.5 | 13.8 | 0.4 | 64 |
| 111. Black currants (Munakka) | 18.4 | 2.7 | 0.5 | 75.2 | 1.0 | 316 |
| 112. Dates, fresh | 59.2 | 1.2 | 0.4 | 33.8 | 3.7 | 144 |
| 113. Figs (Anjeer) | 88.1 | 1.3 | 0.2 | 7.6 | 2.2 | 37 |
| 114. Grapes | 79.2 | 0.5 | 0.3 | 16.5 | 2.9 | 751 |
| 115. Guava | 81.7 | 0.9 | 0.3 | 11.2 | 5.2 | 51 |
| 116. Jackfruit (kathal) | 76.2 | 1.9 | 0.1 | 19.8 | 1.1 | 88 |
| 117. Jamun | 83.7 | 0.7 | 0.3 | 14.0 | 0.9 | 62 |
| 118. Lemon | 85.0 | 1.0 | 0.9 | 11.1 | 1.7 | 57 |
| 110. Lichi | 84.1 | 1.1 | 0.2 | 13.6 | 0.5 | 61 |

| Food Stuff | Moisture (g) | Protein (g) | Fat (g) | Carbohydrate (g) | Fibre (g) | Energy (Cal) |
|---|---|---|---|---|---|---|
| 120. Malta | 90.3 | 0.7 | 0.2 | 7.8 | 0.6 | 36 |
| 121. Musambi | 88.4 | 0.8 | 0.3 | 9.3 | 0.5 | 43 |
| 122. Mango | 81.0 | 0.6 | 0.4 | 16.9 | 0.7 | 74 |
| 123. Muskmelon | 95.2 | 0.3 | 0.2 | 3.5 | 0.4 | 17 |
| 124. Water melon | 95.8 | 0.2 | 0.2 | 3.3 | 0.2 | 16 |
| 125. Orange | 87.6 | 0.7 | 0.2 | 10.9 | 0.3 | 48 |
| 126. Papaya | 90.8 | 0.6 | 0.1 | 7.2 | 0.8 | 32 |
| 127. Peaches (Aarhoo) | 86.0 | 1.2 | 0.3 | 10.5 | 1.2 | 50 |
| 128. Pears (Nashpati) | 86.0 | 0.6 | 0.2 | 11.9 | 1.0 | 52 |
| 129. Phalsa | 80.8 | 1.3 | 0.9 | 14.7 | 1.2 | 72 |
| 130. Pineapple | 87.8 | 0. | 0.1 | 10.8 | 0.5 | 46 |
| 131. Plum (Alubokhara) | 86.9 | 0.7 | 0.5 | 11.1 | 0.4 | 52 |
| 132. Pomegranate | 78.0 | 1.6 | 0.1 | 14.5 | 5.1 | 65 |
| 133. Raisins (Kishmish) | 20.2 | 1.8 | 0.3 | 74.6 | 1.1 | 3048 |
| 134. Sapota (chiku) | 73.7 | 0.7 | 1.1 | 21.4 | 2.6 | 98 |
| 135. Seetaphal (sharifa) | 70.5 | 1.6 | 0.4 | 23.5 | 3.1 | 104 |

| Food Stuff | Moisture (g) | Protein (g) | Fat (g) | Carbohydrate (g) | Fibre (g) | Energy (Cal) |
|---|---|---|---|---|---|---|
| 136. Strawberry | 87.8 | 0.7 | 0.2 | 9.8 | 1.1 | 44 |
| 137. Tomato | 94.0 | 0.9 | 0.2 | 3.6 | 0.8 | 20 |
| 138. Zizyphus (ber) | 81.6 | 0.8 | 0.3 | 17.0 | – | 74 |
| **Milk and Milk Products** | | | | | | |
| 139. Milk, Buffalo's | 81.0 | 4.3 | 6.5 | 5.0 | – | 117 |
| 140. Milk, Cow's | 87.5 | 3.2 | 4.1 | 4.4 | – | 67 |
| 141. Milk, Goat's | 86.8 | 3.3 | 4.5 | 4.6 | – | 72 |
| 142. Curd (Cow's milk) | 89.1 | 3.1 | 4.0 | 3.0 | – | 60 |
| 143. Butter milk | 97.5 | 0.8 | 1.1 | 0.5 | – | 15 |
| 144. Sk. milk, Liquid | 92.1 | 2.5 | 0.1 | 4.6 | – | 29 |
| 145. Chenna, Cow's milk | 57.1 | 18.3 | 20.8 | 1.2 | – | 265 |
| 146. Chenna, Buffalo milk | 54.1 | 13.4 | 23.0 | 7.9 | – | 292 |
| 147. Khoya (Buffalo milk) | 30.6 | 14.6 | 31.2 | 20.5 | – | 421 |
| 148. Khoya (cow milk) | 25.2 | 20.0 | 25.9 | 24.9 | – | 413 |

| Food Stuff | Moisture (g) | Protein (g) | Fat (g) | Carbohydrate (g) | Fibre (g) | Energy (Cal) |
|---|---|---|---|---|---|---|
| 149. Skimmed milk powder (cow's milk) | 4.1 | 38.0 | 0.1 | 51.0 | – | 357 |
| 150. Whole milk powder (cows' milk) | 3.5 | 25.8 | 26.7 | 38.0 | – | 497 |
| **Fats and Oils** | | | | | | |
| 151. Butter | 19.0 | – | – | 81.0 | – | 729 |
| 152. Ghee/Oils | – | – | 100.0 | – | – | 900 |
| **Sugars** | | | | | | |
| 153. Sugar | 0.4 | 0.1 | – | 99.4 | – | 398 |
| 154. Honey | 20.6 | 0.3 | – | 79.5 | – | 319 |
| 155. Jaggery | 3.9 | 0.4 | 0.1 | 95.0 | – | 383 |
| 156. Sago | 12.2 | 0.2 | 0.2 | 87.1 | – | 351 |

**Source:** Nutritive value of Indian Foods, NIN, Indian Council of Medical Research.

# INDEX

D



E



F



G



H

## O



## P, Q



## R



## S



## T